sell / dup

3
14

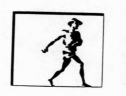

Other books by Dan Georgakas:

RED SHADOWS
THE BROKEN HOOP
DETROIT: I DO MIND DYING
  (with Marvin Surkin)
IN FOCUS: A GUIDE TO USING FILMS
  (with Linda Blackaby and Barbara Margolis)

THE
METHUSELAH
FACTORS

Strategies for a Long and Vigorous Life

DAN GEORGAKAS

SIMON AND SCHUSTER
NEW YORK

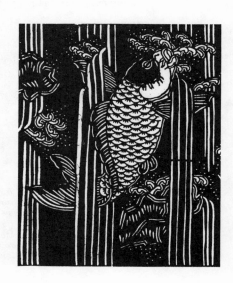

Published by Simon and Schuster
A Division of Gulf & Western Corporation
Simon & Schuster Building
Rockefeller Center
1230 Avenue of the Americas
New York, New York 10020
SIMON AND SCHUSTER and colophon
are trademarks of Simon & Schuster
Designed by Edith Fowler
Photo Editor: Vincent Virga
Manufactured in the United States of America

10   9   8   7   6   5   4   3   2   1

Library of Congress Cataloging in Publication Data

Georgakas, Dan.
    The Methuselah factors.

    Bibliography: p.
    Includes index.
    1. Longevity. I. Title.
QP85.G43   612'.68   80-18609
ISBN 0-671-24064-1
"Desirable Weight Tables for Men and Women," pub-
lished 1959 by the Metropolitan Life Insurance Company,
are used herein by courtesy of the Metropolitan Life
Insurance Company.
The photograph "Grandma Moses at Her Painting Table"
is copyright © 1955 by Grandma Moses Properties Co.,
New York. Used by permission.

To Judy Janda

ACKNOWLEDGMENTS

I thank the long-living people who have generously shared their experiences with me. I especially thank E. W. Salter, who taught me so much about life after 85.

I thank Rhoda Weyr and Alice Mayhew for making it possible for me to realize a boyhood dream of traveling to longevous places. I thank the hundreds of specialists from whose work I've drawn—particularly: A. Ross Eckler for his assistance on American centenarians, Richard Mazess and Sylvia H. Forman for providing materials on Vilcabamba, John Clark for reading the chapter on Hunza and offering detailed criticism, A. Campbell Errol and Stanley Craske for sharing their historical knowledge of Norfolk, Zhores Medvedev for reading the material on the U.S.S.R., Arlene Hoffman and Peter Lubalin for giving me an orientation to Soviet Georgia, Reso Katchelavo for his assistance in Abkhasia, and Shoto Gogoghian for sharing his expertise.

I thank the staffs of the library of the British Museum, the Brooklyn Library (Main Branch), the Library of Congress, and the New York Medical Library and other specialized departments of the New York Public Library. Without those resources and the social forces which support them, this work could not have been done.

I thank the following for reading my manuscript, providing photographs, and assisting my research effort: Melanie Wallace, Peter Pappas, Leonard Rubenstein, Marina Kasdaglis, Deborah Shaffer, Barbara Margolis, Yannis Iordanides, Gary Crowdus, and Rita Arditti. I thank my Soviet friends for accompanying me into the Abkhasian countryside.

I thank Ernest G. Nassar for providing material and offering advice. Long ago, he began to make me familiar with the problems I have dealt with under the heading of "The Toxic Society." As always, he has been the most supportive of friends.

And I thank Judy Janda for her encouragement, her enthusiasm, her photographs, and her editing. My research in the Soviet Union would not have been nearly so productive without her participation. My text would not be accessible or as attractive without her counsel through every stage of development. May she live to be older than Grandma Filkins!

CONTENTS

INTRODUCTION

Before writing had been invented, the Babylonian storytellers sang of the hero Gilgamesh who, when he discovered that only the gods are permitted immortality, sought to be as healthy as a youth all the days of his life. After many tests of his valor, the secret of long life was revealed to him by the Old Man of the Mountain, who spoke of a fragrant plant that looked like a buckthorn and pricked like a rose. The Old Man confided that the plant grew at the bottom of the world's deepest sea, and "If anyone comes into possession of this plant, he can, by tasting it, regain his youth."[1] In time, Gilgamesh was able to locate the fragrant buckthorn rose, but before he could benefit from its rejuvenating powers, it was stolen from him by a serpent seeking a new skin.

Rare is the individual who has not sympathized with Gilgamesh's quest. Whatever the religious or scientific orientation of the day, the human imagination has always been tantalized by the idea of finding a means for the prolongation of life. Each generation has been intrigued by the existence of centenarians and has asked the same basic questions. What is the reason some persons are so much more durable than the rest of humankind? Can emulating the behavior of centenarians help others to reach 100? Is it true that some centenarians have lived more than a hundred and twenty years? What, if any, are the biological limits to human life?

Complicating the consideration of such questions are the hoaxes, swindles, exaggerations, and wishful thinking that are endemic to the subject of long life. The man claiming to be 130 yet looking and acting half that age all too often has no secret to impart other than that he is lying. Fraudulent claims of every kind bedevil all serious inquiries into the means of attaining long life, yet since the end of the nineteenth century reliable data have begun to emerge from the previously impenetrable scramble of fact and fable. The oldest of the documentable old have been systematically identified and their lives rigorously examined.

This work has revealed that most centenarians have a number of shared characteristics. Not surprisingly, this distinctive longevity profile also occurs among the vast majority of people who live to be at least 90, and it is consistent with the most advanced theories of aging and health. The plan of this book is to determine the specifics of the longevity profile and to use them as a basis for formulating a practical longevity agenda. While no health program could ever be a guaranteed formula for reaching 100, an agenda based on the lives of tens of thousands of long-living people is among the more rational approaches available for those who wish to extend the vigor and duration of their lives beyond the usual statistical expectations.

Prior to examining longevity data, it is instructive to review the methods that have repeatedly been suggested as ways of preventing or delaying aging. Most first appeared in the context of fantastic adventures involving the physical courage and spiritual testing of heroic individuals. Although simplistic in their exact prescriptions, many of the stories popularized ideas still considered to have some validity. Building on categories found in Gerald J. Gruman's *History of Ideas About the Prolongation of Life*, it is possible to see that longevity has usually been associated with one or more of the following: magical substances, sacred places, golden ages, complex regimens, and immutable fates.[2]

By far the most prevalent ideas focus on magical substances. Among the most ancient of these are Gilgamesh's undersea plant, Hebraic manna, Iranian haoma, Chinese peaches of immortality, and Indian soma. Other Indian tales dating to at least 700 B.C. describe a Pool of Youth—an idea repeated in sun-drenched Arabia in the form of a Well of Life said to exist in the oasis of El Hidr. Ssu-ma Ch'ien (156–87 B.C.), a Chinese precursor of European alchemists, theorized that mercury compounds might prolong life. That began tales of a long line of magical substances with a base in precious metals or minerals. Throughout the European Middle Ages there were searches for ambrosia, and in the New World rediscovered by Columbus, the Native Americans spoke of a Fountain of Youth hidden in the Florida peninsula and a life-extending octli plant that grew in the Andes.

The earliest magical substances tended to be immersed in religious lore, either as the temptations of evil supernatural forces or as a special boon of the most kindly gods. In time, the magical substances acquired a more scientific nomenclature, becoming, among other things, vitamins, enzymes, hormones, and trace elements. More recently, the magical substance has been a synthetic laboratory product or, at the other extreme, a rediscovered folk remedy involving a rare root or herb. What distinguishes all of these substances—aside from the fact that none of them has been proved to promote longevity unaided—is that they are relatively effortless to use. As with Alice in her Wonderland who drank a potion or nibbled a cake to be instantly short or instantly tall, long life is thought to be a simple matter of sipping, chewing, bathing in, injecting, or swallowing the right magical substance.

Closely associated with the idea of a magical substance is the belief that there is a specially favored earthly habitat where longevity is the norm. This place may be where the magical substance abounds, or it may have the "perfect" human environment. Rather than being at the center of civilization, the terrestial paradise is usually located beyond the farthest boundaries of the known world, a place only the boldest would dare seek. Indian myths spoke of the far-off land of Uttarakuru where the magic tree of life grew. Blessed isles figured in the mythology of Japan, Iran, and the Teutonic tribes. Some cultures had a variety of sacred places. The ever-inventive ancient Greeks had three at various extremities of their world: one high in the mountains of Asia Minor, another in the interior of Ethiopia, and a third on the island or continent beyond the Strait of Gibraltar. The more domesticated the surface of the earth has become, the deeper into jungles and the higher into mountains the sacred places have receded.

A variation of the theme of the sacred place is the legend of a sacred time when the human race enjoyed incredible life-spans. One Roman writer described a lost epoch in which childhood alone lasted a hundred years. Polynesian cultures believed in similar golden ages. And the legendary 969-year-old Methuselah was simply the longest-living of a whole line of longevous antediluvian Hebrews. Bypassing the unanswerable question of how "years" of the long-living epochs were calculated, most golden ages occurred in a period when the human race was thought to be in high favor with the divine forces that guide existence. Since that time, the race had strayed from prescribed moral, dietary, sexual, and social teachings. The consequence of this disobedience was a shorter and more painful time on earth. The only way to restore spiritual harmony and possibly earn divine forgiveness is through a total reformation of self and society, to be achieved through a complex regimen that rigidly controls all facets of behavior.

The reverse of the lost-age coin is the hope that a complex regimen is the means for attaining an unprecedented utopia. An ancient if extreme example of this idea is found in a specific school of Taoists. Its monks combined breathing techniques, dietary principles, specific medicines, regular gymnastics, and spiritual exercises with a sexual discipline in which monks learned to retain their semen even after ejaculation had begun. This system, requiring a lifetime to master, was thought to lead to various planes of enlightenment, culminating in an immortal physical body which the spirit could inhabit or abandon at will. Although most complex regimens do not, like that of these Taoists, consciously exclude half the species or promise corporeal immortality, the regimens demand a total commitment in which life increasingly becomes devoted to the prolongation, enrichment, or surpassing of itself.

The worst aspect of the complex regimens is that individuals must relinquish a large amount of actual present time in the effort to gain an undeterminable amount of added future time. Any regimen that so mortgages and monopolizes the present is further suspect because most longevous people have not lived in such a fashion. More often than not, the manner of their life has been within the norms of their culture, and quite a few of them have been perceived by contemporaries as exemplary citizens. In contrast, the complex regimens often remove people from society or involve them in cultish behavior. While some of the specific techniques of complex regimens can be incorporated into a more rational approach to life extension, none of the regimens has ever demonstrated that it can produce unusual health or longevity. Utopia never materializes. But like the concept of a lost golden age, the notion of a complex regimen is valid in its insistence that rather than a single longevity secret, there is a complex of longevity factors. Unless each of the factors is represented in a conscious longevity agenda, the prospects of unusually long life are greatly diminished.

Lastly, there is the view that longevity is a matter largely beyond human manipulation. Those who favor an immutable-fate approach range from gamblers who believe long life is primarily a matter of luck to determinists who ascribe it to unalterable genetic inheritance. The gamblers often speak of the futility of planning for longevity because one might die from an accident. This overlooks the fact that in a nation like the United States less than 5 percent of the entire adult population will die through accidents, while more than 70 percent will die from diseases greatly influenced by life-style.[3] Gamblers delight in speaking of some 95-year-old obese drunkard who chain-smokes cigarettes and has never exercised. Such characters may exist, but they are only slightly less rare than unicorns. Like the roulette addict, the gambler is banking on luck in a game in which the long-run odds of winning are nil.

The genetic argument is another matter. The question is not whether inheritance is a longevity factor, but to what extent, and whether the inheritance is as immutable as was once believed. One important touchstone is that although inherited diseases and physiological weaknesses can have a definite adverse affect on longevity prospects, to date no genetic factor that positively promotes long life has been discovered. However, since longevous women far outnumber longevous men in every society, the possibility of a linkage between longevity and the genes that determine sex cannot be ruled out.[4] Other more observable, but less important, genetically influenced characteristics that affect longevity would include overall body size, the basal metabolic rate, and various chemical idiosyncrasies.

Theoretically, the genetic code determines the outer limit for any given individual's development, while the quality of the environment determines how much of the potential capacity is actually realized. Present medical knowledge indicates that the body is programmed to endure, if it is not abused, for more than a century. Were we at a stage where large numbers of people were becoming centenarians, determining the feasibility of genetic reprogramming would be a top longevity priority. As this is not the case, achieving the programmed genetic limits remains a reasonable objective.

What the upper genetic limits are returns us to the search for the oldest of the old. An ideal age verification would involve several independently arrived-at proofs occurring over a period of time in a logical sequence consistent with established statistical and scientific principles. The first chapter of this book begins with an examination of the evidence offered for the oldest documented centenarian, Delina Filkins (1815–1928), and proceeds to consider historical and contemporary claims that others have lived much longer. The historical review concentrates most heavily on the period for which at least some documentation is available and culminates in the investigation of centenarian claims for specific national groups and geographical locations. The most celebrated of these originate in the Caucasus, where, during the 1970s, hundreds of persons claimed to be over 120. Of equal interest are similar supercentenarian claims for the Vilcabamba Valley of the Ecuadorian Andes and for the Hunza Valley of the western Himalayas. Also investigated are the more modest but still extraordinary age claims for the Tarahumara Indians of the Sierra Madre range in Mexico, the village of Upper Sheringham in Great Britain, and mountain peoples of Eastern Europe and Turkey.

Just as important as age claims for individuals or regions are claims made for unusual physical vigor among the very old. The wisdom of the oft-quoted epigram that we must add life to our years as well as years to our life should be self-evident. Few would want to accumulate calendar years consisting of prolonged infirmity and discomfort. As will be seen, many of the investigations that debunk extraordinary age claims confirm the reality of extremely vigorous sep-

tuagenarians and octogenarians and relatively active nonagenarians. These findings correlate with work done by
physical-fitness experts in the United States which demonstrates that the vitality commonly associated with a healthy
40-year-old can be enjoyed in one's 70s and 80s.[5] Whether or
not the total life-span exceeds one hundred years, this means
that most people can add from two to three decades to what is
now considered a prime time of life.

Available studies devoted to every aspect of aging are
legion, yet there is a serious communication gap between
historians, anthropologists, physicians, chemists, and other
specialists. It often seems that all the separate items needed
for an effective longevity agenda have been identified long
ago but remain scattered in disconnected segments, much
like the pieces of a disassembled jigsaw puzzle. A case in
point is Hunza. Although it is usually depicted as an area
nearly inaccessible to visitors and for which there is a paucity
of information, there are, in fact, literally scores of books,
journals, chapter entries, and diary notes by visitors going
back over a century and commenting upon every facet of
Hunzakut society. Fitting the pieces together provides a most
coherent and credible portrait of Hunzakut longevity. Likewise, piecing together the longevity knowledge scattered
through various disciplines produces a most lucid account of
how the oldest of the old have lived and the best ways to
emulate them.

In order to facilitate comparison of work done in different time periods and nations by people using various
methodologies, terminology throughout this book has been
standardized as much as possible. Individuals from 60 to 79
will be referred to as being in their late maturity; individuals
from 80 to 89 as old; individuals from 90 to 109 as longevous;
individuals from 110 to 114 as superlongevous; and individuals claiming more than 115 years as supercentenarians.[6]
References to the developed world indicate the United States,
Canada, Japan, Europe, and all areas of the Soviet Union.

Finally, no proposed longevity project would be complete

without reference to the various artificial means for the extension of life now being researched throughout the world. Some successes are anticipated before the end of the present century; and it is conceivable that eventually a long series of antiaging interventions could carry life-spans to the years of Methuselah and even to the threshold of physical immortality, the lost hope of Gilgamesh. Scientists usually like to discourage the more sensational ramifications of antiaging research by stating that their efforts are only one more step in the process that brought about blood transfusions, pacemakers, organ transplants, wonder drugs, and other weapons in the life-sustaining arsenal. Yet, barring unforeseen difficulties, we appear to be on the brink of a longevity explosion in which a hundredth birthday will cease to be a novelty. It is possible that people already alive may become the first fully documented supercentenarians.

Dazzling as the longevity prospects of the near future are, the longevity agenda identified in the pages that follow is independent of drugs, procedures, and other means not presently available. The program has four major goals. The first is to improve immediate general health. The second is to surpass the average life-span. The third is to achieve a vigorous longevity. The fourth is to extend life beyond one hundred at a time when new knowledge may make our present expectations seem as limited as the twenty-to-thirty-year average life-spans of the Roman Empire.

Part One

THE LONGEVITY PROFILE

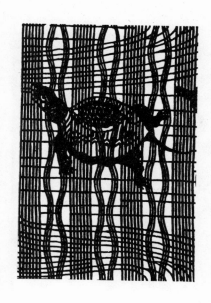

1

THE OLDEST OF THE OLD

> No single subject is more obscured
> by vanity, deceit, falsehood, and de-
> liberate fraud than the extremes of
> human longevity.
>
> —*Guinness Book of World Records*

Delina Filkins of Herkimer County, New York, who lived
from May 4, 1815, to December 4, 1928, is the longest-lived
documented individual known. Shirali Mislimov of Barzavu,
Azerbaijan, who died in 1973 at the reputed age of approximately 170, is the longest-living undocumented person
claimed by responsible authorities during modern times.
Numerous other individuals, recently deceased or still living,
have claimed life-spans exceeding Filkins' 113 years and 214
days but less than Mislimov's alleged seventeen decades.
Somewhere in this group is the outer boundary of achieved
human longevity.

The age of "Grandma" Filkins was verified by A. Ross
Eckler, who was able to trace her life from 1850 to 1925 in
the national and state census records found in the Herkimer
County Courthouse. This census material established that
from 1850 onward, information as to the age of Mrs. Filkins

(nee Ecker), the ages of her children, and the age of her husband remained constant. The ages proceeded one year at a time, and subsequent information concerning Filkins was internally consistent. Interviews with her descendants established that for all her life she had lived within a ten-mile radius of the family's dairy farm and had been active in its extensive cheese business. Her father had been longevous (97), and her mother had reached late maturity (73). To the end of her life, despite some deafness, Filkins retained a keen interest in world affairs and enjoyed reading. She was said to be fond of bragging that the only medicines she had ever taken were "sleeping herbs."[1]

Confidence in Filkins' age is bolstered by the fact that in her own day, while her age was duly noted in the local papers and she enjoyed limited regional fame, she never sought to profit from her years. She was a relatively obscure person at the time of her death; her major obituary appeared in the *Herkimer Evening Telegram*, and the two known portraits of her hang in the Van Hornesville Central School and in the Canajoharie Library and Art Gallery. Until A. Ross Eckler presented her documentation to the *Guinness Book of World Records*, Grandma Filkins was just another frontier character, and to this day there is no national or regional celebration of her unique status.

Nor has the "discoverer" of Grandma Filkins sought any personal limelight. A. Ross Eckler, who earned a Ph.D. from Princeton in the field of mathematics, has been employed as a statistician by New Jersey Bell Telephone for more than a quarter of a century. Eckler has traced the genealogy of his own family and done numerous longevity studies as a hobby. By scrutinizing census data, Eckler has discovered that many Americans seeking notoriety advanced their ages fifteen to twenty years for every ten years of the census, with the inflation usually commencing around age 70. He believes that all of the unresolved American claims for longevity greater than that of Grandma Filkins are invalid and that many are outright deceptions. Since there is an impressive array of tax, legal, and census documentation on three levels of government, it is difficult to believe that many Americans, particularly anyone living more than one hundred years, could escape all official notice. Eckler's own interest in Filkins was providential. His family happened to have a farm in Herkimer, and he had been intrigued by stories about the local centenarian told by his own longevous relatives.

The Filkins claim is satisfactory from a mathematical standpoint as well. Her life exceeded that of the previously recognized oldest person by only eighty-six days, a development quite in line with statistical probability. If someone is ever proved to have outlived Filkins, that new record will likely conform to what is now an established pattern: the newest documented outer boundary of age exceeding the previous one by a short period, with a number of additional persons added to the list of those who have lived beyond 110, 111, and 112, respectively.

The precedent for using mathematical probabilities and governmental records was set by the Englishman William J. Thoms, who wrote about centenarians in the latter half of the nineteenth century, publishing his landmark *The Longevity of Man* in 1873.[2] Throughout his work, Thoms insisted on standards that have since been accepted as the basis for age verification. Thoms, who was a deputy librarian in the British House of Lords, had originally been intrigued by three British subjects who had been claimed as supercentenarians: the Countess of Desmond (140), Thomas Parr (152), and Henry Jenkins (169).

Thoms reasoned that even the humblest Briton would have had a difficult time escaping all official documentation. Since 1538, every parson, vicar, and curate had been required by law to keep a record of all christenings, weddings, and funerals in his parish. To mandatory parish records could be added tax rolls, land contracts, court proceedings, military lists, and other documents. During times more recent to Thoms's own era, there were records kept by life-insurance firms that were especially concerned about the correct age and identity of their clients. Thoms began the test of a claim by trying to find a parish record and continued it by looking for other materials that described the same person.

Certain bases for fraud were found to recur. Entries in the family Bible often did not jibe with baptismal and marriage records. Frequently, this was due to related persons who had identical names or occurred because many parents, anticipating that one or more of their offspring would die during childhood, gave exactly the same name to two or more siblings. Another finding was that the claimed birth date and the written baptismal date could be separated by a gap of many years. This was explained as a function of the parents putting off the ritual until the child understood its significance or as a result of financial or social considerations. Suspiciously, the highest age claims were often found in conjunction with these delayed baptisms. Claimants also offered news clippings as verification when the story only repeated verbatim what they had told an obliging correspondent. The "proof" was their own word. The internal details of most stories fell apart under the mildest scrutiny, as the deceptions were primarily good-natured boasting rather than swindles.

At a certain point in his labors, Thoms began to doubt if anyone had ever turned 100; but gradually, from various sources, authentic case histories began to accumulate. The major breakthrough in verification came from Canada, where Dr. Joseph Tache, Dominion Statistician at Ottawa, undertook a study of 421 centenarian claims made between 1609 and 1876. Finding that it was extremely difficult to get reliable data on those born outside Canada, Tache had narrowed his list to the 82 who were native-born. Of these 82, he determined that 9 were valid centenarians. Among those 9 was Pierre Joubert, a French Canadian lumberjack who had lived from July 15, 1701, to November 16, 1814. His 113 years and 124 days was to stand as the longest documented life-span until the verification of Grandma Filkins'. Unlike so many others who proved to be liars, Joubert had shunned all publicity and had believed himself to be younger than his actual years. His age, however, was verified through church records found by parish priests working under the direction of Dr. Tache and Abbé Cyprien Tanguay, Canada's first genealogist.

Claims for the 3 fabled supercentenarians of the British Isles proved to be of much less substance. The case of the Countess of Desmond (1464–1604) was the weakest. A long-living Countess of Desmond had existed, but she had never claimed to be a supercentenarian and most likely was not aware of the myths surrounding her age. Testimony that purported to be firsthand fell under the weight of impossible internal contradictions. The final explanation for the supposed supercentenarianism was that the lives of 2 or 3 women who had borne the title had been grafted to create 1 fictitious superwoman.

On the surface, the tale of Thomas Parr (1483–1635) seemed to have more merit. Charles I had received him at court, and Sir William Harvey, the physician who discovered the circulation of blood, had performed an autopsy on him which was widely interpreted as having verified his great age. Parr's legend included the belief that he had been extraordinarily endowed sexually. In 1588, at the alleged age of 105, he had been ordered to do public penance for indecent sexual overtures to a woman, and seventeen years later, at the alleged age of 122, he had married for a second time.

Researching the story with his usual skepticism, Thoms became convinced that it was the invention of the Earl of Arundel, a courtier who wanted to regain lost favor with the sovereign, and that Harvey had obliged the Earl because of a personal debt. A reading of the actual autopsy report revealed that Harvey had made it clear that he was responsible only for the technical matter and that all else was "furnished by the person who accompanied Parr to London."[3] That person, of course, was the Earl of Arundel. Except for a whimsical comment that the stories of Parr's sexual powers had a physiological basis, the physician's report was straightforward, concluding that Parr had indeed been a very old man.

Moving from Harvey's autopsy, Thoms delved into the matter of leases at the Parr cottage and discovered that on one occasion Parr had resorted to elaborate trickery to retain his right to the cottage and adjoining land. Subsequent research was to discover that 3 Thomas Parrs had lived consecutively at the Parr cottage: a father, his son, and his grandson. Old people who remembered Thomas Parr as being old when they were young likely were thinking of the father or grandfather. Several persons claiming to be Parr's children had substantiated his age with their own word, but they had never presented documentary proof and could not even establish their own relationship to him. Thoms pointed out that according to Parr's own account, all the children of his first marriage had died and the second marriage had been childless.

Other aspects of the Parr legend were that he continued to work in the fields until he was 130, that he enjoyed sexual relations until he was 140, and that he remained vigorous until he left Shropshire to go down to London, where he promptly expired as a result of frantic merrymaking. Investigation turned up a more credible portrait. Several sources agreed that Parr had been blind for at least twenty years, that he was quite frail, and that his memory was so greatly impaired that he could recall only recent events. Recognizing that Parr had probably been longevous, Thoms repeatedly requested surveys of all parish records in the region of Parr's birth. No documentation was forthcoming. The proof of 152 years came to rest solely on the word of a frail, blind, poor old man and the ambitious courtier who had exploited him. Mainly because of the mistaken assumption about Harvey's endorsement, Thomas Parr is still cited as a legitimate or probable supercentenarian in some books that are otherwise quite serious, and his myth is a standby of faddist literature.

The tale of Henry Jenkins (1511–1670) proved to be even

weaker, with the strong possibility that Yorkshire officials had built it up in deliberate rivalry with Parr's earlier claim in Shropshire. Jenkins, who liked to call himself "the oldest man born upon the ruins of the postdiluvian world," was never able to keep his claim consistent. Depending on the occasion, his age went up and down like a yo-yo. One of the proofs his adherents thought strongest was that Jenkins had sworn that he was 157 years old in a court case involving Charles Anthony, a vicar. Yet twelve years later, after his burial, Charles Anthony discreetly listed Jenkins as "a very aged and poore man"[4] in the only parish record found for him. People who spoke up to confirm Jenkins' age were proved to be lying about their own and thus could not have witnessed the events they claimed to have seen.

As with so many undocumented individuals, Jenkins' notoriety began late in life—in this case after the asserted age of 130. This raises the question why he was not famous at 110, or 120, particularly since Thoms had demonstrated that any centenarianism was rare. The answer is self-evident. Like Parr's, Jenkins' claim was based entirely on his word, and like Parr, he was not telling the truth. An aspect of his legend illustrates how tales grow. Alternatingly, Jenkins was said to have been a soldier in the Battle of Flodden, to have taken arrows as a young man to soldiers in the battle, or to have taken arrows as a child to a young man who gave them to the soldiers who fought. Most likely he had heard stories about the battle from his parents or grandparents.

The pattern of deception found in Parr and Jenkins was to be encountered by Thoms many times as he became the first to take issue with how often the most spectacular age claims were found in conjunction with high rates of illiteracy. His doubts were countered with the argument that the simple life of the peasant was more "natural"—a favorite theme of romantics influenced by Jean Jacques Rousseau. Yet throughout Europe, as soon as record keeping with any degree of accuracy was established, the same peasant class that had boasted of longevity developed much shorter life-spans and relatively poor health. In developed nations, education and longevity have had a consistently strong positive correlation.

Thoms concluded that centenarians were something of a biological fluke. He found that in Scotland the legal presumption of the limit of life was one hundred years. For him, this was folk wisdom at its best. He further noted that in Chapter 18, Verse 9 of Ecclesiasticus it was written that "The number of man's days is great if he reaches a hundred years."

Writing twenty years after Thoms, T.E. Young pioneered another method of longevity verifications. The key to his approach is found in the dedication of his book to the Institute of Actuaries, an organization founded in 1848. Young believed the most reliable longevity data could be found in actuarial tables, since the very solvency of powerful insurance companies depended on their accuracy. He noted that firms picked up their clients at a relatively young age, verified that age, and kept track of each person for life. While the clients of nineteenth-century firms were mainly the urban middle class, their statistics provided a guidepost for judging figures applicable to the general population. Confining himself to insurance records, Young established that of 30,000 persons covered by contracts from 1770 to 1890, there were only 22 indisputable centenarians, the oldest of them having lived to 105. Females had outnumbered males by 2 to 1. Using this result and similar data, Young estimated that from 1821 to 1871, when the British population was increasing from 21 to 31 million, there had been 200 to 250 centenarians alive at any given moment. As insurance companies came to embrace more of the population and as census records become more reliable, Young believed longevity verification could approach the accuracy of an exact science.

Young fought against hearsay and flimsy evidence. He wrote that since tombstones usually set forth inflated sentiments and language, the dates carved on them were by no means dependable. He noted that one 78-year-old man had had his age recorded as 708 because the carver was told he was 70 and 8. Young's perusal of historical and medical records led him to conclude that from the thirteenth to the sixteenth century, 70 was usually considered a great age in Britain. Fascinated by the mystery of numbers, he also attempted to deal with antediluvian biblical longevity by speculating as to what might have constituted a year on the basis of a variety of numerical theories. A more practical contribution was his inclusion of specific research used to reach his conclusions.[5] One of his consultants was Dr. G. M. Humphry, professor of surgery at Cambridge. Humphry had examined 900 patients thought to be at least 90 years of age. Of those 900, 52 were believed to be centenarians. The following data for the 36 women and 16 men were recorded:[6]

1. The majority were moderate or light eaters.
2. The majority ate little meat.
3. The majority liked to do outdoor work and rose early.
4. Forty drank alcohol.
5. Few reported having had many illnesses.
6. Forty-four reported they were excellent sleepers, most averaging over eight hours a night for most of their lives.
7. A large percentage claimed to be from long-lived families, although "long-lived" was not carefully defined and not documented.
8. Twelve were firstborn children.
9. Over two-thirds of the women had been married and had raised large families.
10. Ten of the 11 who were over 102 were female, the oldest person being 105.

In the 1930s, Maurice Ernest gave a larger European context to the tradition initiated by Thoms and Young.[7] Surveying historical records from Roman times onward, he was unable to locate a single credible case of any European who had lived as long as Pierre Joubert. What he did find was that monarchs were most enthusiastic about having the oldest specimens of humanity among their subjects, resulting in numerous hoaxes of the Desmond-Parr-Jenkins ilk. An example of this was Drakenberg the Dane, a Scandinavian sailor reputed to have reached 146 (1626–1772). Investigation showed the story to have no foundation.

Nationalism influenced longevity claims in other ways. With the decline of the Ottoman Empire in the late nineteenth century, there were hundreds of supercentenarian claims in the newly independent Balkan states or in regions of the Austro-Hungarian Empire. Like most patriotic lore, the longevity tales were most credible on festive holidays when accompanied by wine, music, and general good feeling. With the establishment of even crude record keeping, these same areas were soon shown to have the poorest health, the lowest average life-spans, and the fewest centenarians in Europe. The scale of falsification was evident in an incident from Bavaria. When the 1871 census turned up 37 centenarian claims, the government made an official inquiry. It was discovered that most of the claimants had not reached 90 and 1 individual proved to be a mere 61. In the final count, there was only 1 genuine centenarian.[8]

In spite of many incidents of this kind, stories of longevity in Eastern and Southern Europe persisted, enhanced by scientists fascinated by what they believed was a link between cultured milk products and long life. Led by the brilliant Eli Metchnikoff, who had discovered the disease-fighting role of phagocytes, they believed that live yogurt bacillus penetrated into the intestinal tract, where it worked against toxins that might poison the body before being released as waste matter. Yogurt experts squabbled over which strain was best and whether a solid or semiliquid form was most advantageous. In addition to the obvious overtones of magical-substance wishful thinking, the theme was given golden-age and sacred-place orchestration by writers who insisted that the peasants represented a purer form of humanity than that found in cities or in Western Europe. Although later studies proved that yogurt bacteria are destroyed by stomach acids, belief in the prolongevous qualities of yogurt has continued.

A more encouraging finding reported by Ernest originated in Scotland, where the Registrar General of Births had decided to examine every centenarian claim made from 1910 to 1932. Involved were 253 females and 48 males, for a total of 301 persons. Ninety-nine claims were inconclusive because of insufficient data. Of the remaining 202 individuals, the remarkably high number of 157 (137 females and 18 males) were found to be telling the truth. The oldest man was 103, and the oldest woman 106 years and 213 days.[9] These findings indicated either a sudden acceleration in longevity since the Thoms-Young period or more accurate recognition of longevity that had existed all along.

Ernest located many other valid centenarians to go along with the Scottish group. Of greatest significance were the proofs found for Mrs. Ann Pouder (over 110), Mrs. Margaret Ann Neve (almost 111), and the Honorable Katherine Plunkett (almost 112). This trio, combined with Joubert, proved that a superlongevous club of 110 plus was indeed a human reality. The sample, it must be stressed, was limited to Anglo-American records (mainly from 1750 onward) and thus represented only a fraction of the human population; and even within this fraction, the number was confined to fully documented individuals.

Unlike his predecessors', Ernest's stated objective was to find the secret of longevity. He was knowledgeable about the medical opinion of his era and studied the biographies of longevous people, particularly those who had written about health. At times, he speculated that if certain physical processes could be understood, the present maximal life-spans could be doubled or even tripled. For practical purposes, however, he believed 120 was the realizable limit of human life. His prescription was:

- Eat frugally.
- Exercise and get plenty of fresh air.
- Choose a congenial occupation.
- Develop a placid or easygoing personality.
- Maintain a high level of personal hygiene.

- Drink wholesome liquids.
- Abstain from stimulants and sedatives.
- Get plenty of rest.
- Have a waste evacuation once a day.
- Live in a temperate climate.
- Enjoy a reasonable sex life.
- Get prompt medical attention in case of illness.

Ernest also reported on some of the hoaxes that had accumulated in the new century. Increasingly, the new sites of longevity were located beyond the Bosporus and involved non-Christian cultures. A typical case was that of Zaro Agha, an illiterate Turkish citizen from Kurdistan. Agha said he was 156 and claimed to have seen Napoleon when the General was residing in Egypt. A theatrical manager arranged for travel documents, and Agha was soon in the United States and Great Britain. While never able to convince researchers of his age, Agha had a brief moment of glory on theatrical stages before returning to Turkey, where he died in obscurity in 1933.[10]

Apparently that was a poor year for supercentenarians, for in May, Li Chung Yun, a Chinese herb seller, was reported by *The New York Times* to have perished at the incredible age of 197.[11] Written with obvious humor (a previous age claim would have made him 256), the story would not be worth citing if it did not involve yet another common magical substance—the rare Oriental herb. In this case, the plant was called fo-ti tien (literal meaning: the elixir of life). Naturally, it could be found only in a difficult-to-reach region. Those who retold the story never explained why the herb was not used by the natives who brought it to Li Chung Yun or why he had withheld his secret from his reported 23 wives and their numerous offspring. Stranger still, the herbs Li Chung Yun sold to others were advertised as being able to extend life to a mere one hundred years. When tested under laboratory conditions, fo-ti tien, like ginseng and other miraculous roots and herbs, was found to have no pro-longevous effects.[12]

A much more substantial claim to long life than that of Li Chung Yun, and easily the best claim currently available that anyone has ever lived longer than Delina Filkins, belongs to Shigechiyo Izumi of Japan, who celebrated his 114th birthday on June 29, 1979, and is alive at the time of this writing. Izumi lives on a tiny island of fisherfolk located just south of the major island of Kyushu. Telephone communication with the registrar of the Isen town office on Tokonushima island, Kagoshima Perfecture, revealed that when the Family Registration Act of Emperor Meiji's government went into effect in 1871, a Shigechiyo Izumi was recorded as having been born on June 29, 1865. Family records, which are meticulously kept in Japan, indicate that the present Shigechiyo Izumi is the 6-year-old of 1871.[13] This evidence has satisfied the Japanese government, the Kyodo News Service, and the *Guinness Book of World Records*.

The major reservation in accepting Izumi as the oldest documented human is that the specifics of his claim have not been verified by professional researchers. This is an important consideration, as such investigators have shown in other claims of extreme age that although the submitted documentation was authentic, it had been applied to the wrong individual. The Japanese Ministry of Health and Welfare has provided this author with a thumbnail sketch of Izumi which includes the information that his father died three months after Izumi's birth and that his mother died three months later. The child was then cared for and raised by an uncle. Izumi was wed in 1904 at the age of 39, but there were no children of the marriage until 1916 at which time a son, Suehiro, was born. The infant was to die one year later. In 1917, when Izumi was 52, his first daughter , Yoshi, was born. She was to die at 19. In 1930 Izumi became a porter at Port Kaura, and he held that job until 1951. His wife, Miya, died in 1956 after fifty-two years of marriage, and in 1965 Izumiu received a congratulatory letter and a silver cup from Prime Minister Sato to celebrate his 100th birthday.

The communication from the Ministry and newspaper stories indicate that at age 114, Izumi gets up at about eight in the morning and goes for a walk with his dog after breakfast. At night, he drinks a pint of warm *shocku* (potato liquor) with his meal, likes to watch television, and goes to bed at about nine. He is described as a moderate smoker and states that he has never worried too much. He has no dietary peculiarities, but prefers fish and vegetables to meat. The Ministry states that Izumi's blood pressure, eyesight, hearing, and internal organs are "normal," without indicating on what criteria the evaluation is based. News reports describe him as vigorous.

Izumi's celebrity happens to cap a more-than-decade-long centenarian boom in the Japanese media. In addition to reporting on the nearly 1,000 known Japanese centenarians, the media have given extensive, if somewhat uncritical, coverage to various longevity claims around the world. Izumi may indeed be the age claimed for him, but even in his summary available biography are several areas that beg for clarification. The death of both parents before he was 7 months old and the fact that he was born before the Family Registration Act went into effect make it imperative that great attention be paid to detail to determine that there was no mistaken identity at a very early age. The twelve-year gap between his marriage to Miya and the time their first children were born is somewhat unusual and should also be investigated. Another area requiring scrutiny is the nature of the work involved in the porter's job begun at age 65 and held until age 86. The "normal" health readings are most suspicious, in that loss of efficiency is observable in all humans as they age and should be especially apparent in the longest-living human of all time. None of these questions about the data available on Izumi are insurmountable, but his age cannot be considered verified until professionals have compiled family genealogies, cross-checked the records, assessed his health by objective criteria, and otherwise clarified the details of his biography.

Another intriguing claim for extraordinary age comes from Mali. The story was brought to European attention through the work of pioneer visual anthropologist Jean Rouch, most of whose films have dealt with traditional cultures found within contemporary African societies. In 1969 while working on a project, he was informed that Anai Dollo, the village elder of Bongo, had died. An unusual funeral was being prepared, for not only had Anai Dollo been head of the Society of Masks, he was believed to be over 122 years of age.[14] Dollo belonged to the Auru subgroup of the Dogon people, and one of his tribe's most sacred rites is celebrated at sixty-year intervals. He had been present at three of these: once as a baby, once as a mature adult of 60, and two and half years before Rouch's visit as the village elder.

There is little doubt concerning the accuracy of the sixty-year cycles. Genealogy in the tribe is kept by oral historians noted for their precision, and Dollo had become such a highly respected member of the Auru that unless there was a fraud in progress throughout the tribe, any switch of identity would have to have occurred extremely early in his life. The possibility of a hoax was further discounted by the fact that although his people considered him to be extraordinarily old, neither they, Rouch, nor the Mali government knew that if his story was true, he had lived a full eight years longer than the oldest documented person. Rouch's interest at the time had been in photographing a spectacular funeral which involved singing, dancing, recitations, and mock battles.

The oral tradition by which Dollo's age was preserved has proved that it can be as accurate as written records. Researchers in North America found, for example, that the individual recollections of Indian warriors bound by strict tribal and fraternal codes of honor were far more accurate when citing battle casualties and other war details than were the written accounts of cavalry officers or reporters seeking to make an impression on their military superiors or the general public. The African oral tradition has proved to be of equal strength and veracity. Dollo's age claim reflects the word of an entire people, rather than one person.

The dating for the rituals appears to be on firm ground too. The Dogon, who have long been the favorites of French anthropologists because of their sense of order, style, and precision, have a sophisticated astronomy. When questioned about the possibility that the sixty-year cycle might be off, Rouch thought it was extremely unlikely and noted that Europeans had been present at the ritual in 1907 and that the next cycle had taken place in 1967 right on schedule. There was no reason to doubt that the earlier one had occurred in 1847. Rouch also thought it unlikely that there had been any falsification of Anai's age. He emphasized the Dogon passion for exact calculations and the regularity with which the tribe's history was publicly recounted. Just as noteworthy in his opinion was the respect the Dogon showed to the old. If persons became so feeble that they could not take care of themselves, they were placed on a platform in the vestibule of the family lodge. Everyone going in and coming out was required to speak with the oldster, maintaining his or her connection to daily life and preventing any sense of loneliness or abandonment. Dollo, blind for over two years and quite frail, had been treated in this manner.

Speculation on the longevity of Africans fed an allied interest in the United States during the 1950s and '60s when there was a rash of stories about black centenarians who had been slaves. The *Ebony* magazine story about 114-year-old Henry Hudson who had spoken with Abraham Lincoln was typical.[15] Popularizers advanced the notion that a black physical elite may have been created because the horrors of the slave trade had killed off the weaker men and women en route from Africa and the rigors of slavery itself had bred exceptional strength. It was further argued that slaves had eaten simple, wholesome food and they had not been under the stress of economic worries. For whites, there was certainly more than a little racism in the idea that people constantly in fear of being sold or physically mistreated could live without stress. Like that of the rich city-bred Europeans who idolized the noble peasantry, the American idea of longevous ex-slaves made it seem that slavery, like serfdom, had not been without its advantages. For blacks, there was some psychological pleasure in believing that the slaves had outlived their masters.

Investigation of plantation registers and postemancipation census records soon proved most claims to be false. More difficult were cases in which the claimant deliberately threw off the researchers with false information so that no documentation could be located. The most famous of these was that of Charlie Smith, who told a 1955 Social Security official that he had been born in Liberia in 1842. In one story he had been lured aboard a slave ship through false promises, and in another he had been knocked from his bicycle and kidnapped. A man of considerable charm, Charlie told his stories well, aided, perhaps, by his experiences as a carnival worker. By 1979, now claiming to be 137 years old, Smith had become a celebrity, his life extolled in a filmed docudrama and his words reproduced in numerous newspaper and magazine articles. Most gerontologists, however, had never accepted his claim because of the inconsistencies, historical errors, and improbabilities found in his many public statements. They were not surprised when a researcher associated with the *Guinness Book of World Records* found a Florida marriage license which showed that Smith had added a whopping thirty-three years to his true age. He had become a genuine centenarian only in 1975. Smith died in October of 1979 without ever being told that his true age had been discovered.

The remaining unresolved ex-slave supercentenarian claims are quite doubtful. The researcher of Delina Filkins has found only two with partial documentation. One of them is that of Mark Thrash, who died in 1943, and had claimed to be 123 years old. The 1900 federal census shows a Mark Thrash in the Crawfish Springs Militia District who claims to have been born on December 18, 1822. Whether it is indeed the same man, and a genuine claim, has not been confirmed. Nor have any other Thrash records been located. The second former slave of note is Martha Graham, who died in 1959 at the reputed age of 117 or 118. The 1900 census for Cumberland County, North Carolina, shows a Martha Graham married to a Henry Graham, and the same family unit appears in the 1880 count. The ages found in the two censuses would have made Graham 116 years old at her death if it is the same Martha. No other record for her has been found.[16]

Mark Thrash and Martha Graham notwithstanding, the known life-spans of blacks in the United States do not augur well for the existence of superlongevity among them. Blacks have consistently had poorer health and lower life expectancy than the general population. Only since the 1940s have they begun to approach its average life-span. Despite rapid gains, equalization will probably not occur until the end of the twentieth century. The depressed living conditions and economic exploitation suffered by most blacks is more than sufficient explanation for this phenomenon, and those factors are compounded by the circumstance that until the 1940s most blacks lived in the South, which traditionally has had the nation's poorest health. Of course, black centenarians do exist; Charlie Smith was one of them; but they do not seem to live as long or to appear in as large a percentage as the national average.

Another population reputed to be superlongevous is that found in the Caucasus. Although longevity research in the region dates back to at least the early 1900s, the problem of age verification has been formidable. Under the tsars the region was administrated indifferently, and its people left illiterate. When inhabitants were asked their ages, they might respond with reckonings in other than the Christian calendar. As in Central Asia, they might refer to twelve-year cycles, each named after an animal. Having been born in the Year of the Bear could indicate 1880 or 1892 or 1904. Of the minimal records kept by the tsarist bureaucracy or religious authorities, few survived the fighting associated with the Revolution, the civil war, and World War II.

Confronted by this lack of documentation, contemporary

Soviet researchers have had to rely heavily on detailed life histories obtained through personal interviews. Each centenarian is asked to recall his or her age at the time of important historical events. The responses are then compared with whatever records exist, the testimony of family members, and the histories of other persons living in the area. Clearly, such a method would be subject to error with even the most highly trained personnel. The problem is more severe in the U.S.S.R. because many of the old people do not understand Russian and it is not always possible to find a person skilled in the local language or dialect who also is professionally competent in taking oral histories. Untrained interpreters or untrained interviewers often must determine if a war in the east is the one needed to confirm a fabulous age or if a particular Year of the Bear is really 1880 and not 1892 or 1904. Respect for the word of the old, ethnic chauvinism, and plain wishful thinking have probably fostered more distortions than deliberate chicanery has. Aware of this situation, the Soviet authorities have issued a manual to interviewers which runs to 272 pages. The sheer size of the tome is a good indication of the magnitude of their concern.

In spite of their reputation for secrecy, the Soviets have been fairly generous in allowing foreigners to interview their centenarians. Particularly after 1970, when announcement of some 500 supercentenarians claims elicited worldwide awe at just the time when détente made travel much easier, many foreign reporters and scientists visited the longevous regions. Among the most important American researchers were Dr. Sula Benet, an anthropologist employed by the Institute for the Study of Man and by Hunter College—City University of New York, and Dr. Alexander Leaf, a medical doctor on the staff of Boston General Hospital and the faculty of the Harvard Medical School. After several trips to the Caucasus, the Russian-speaking Benet enthusiastically endorsed the Soviet findings. A somewhat more skeptical Leaf, who had studied longevity in the U.S.S.R., Ecuador, and Hunza for the National Geographic Society, was also impressed. Acceptance of this kind was characteristic of most Western observers.

In 1976, a populist twist was given to the centenarian craze by an advertising agency representing the Dannon yogurt company. Soviet cooperation was secured to film a series of commercials featuring officially verified Georgian centenarians and supercentenarians, who compared American yogurt with their own homemade variety. As a result of the exceptionally clever and entertaining advertisements, which appeared in magazines and on television, elements of Georgian folklore merged with American pop culture.

The major dissenting voice in the longevity euphoria belonged to geneticist Zhores A. Medvedev. Although of Russian ethnicity, Medvedev had been born in Tbilisi, Georgia, and had traveled throughout the Caucasus. Medvedev had been trained by the Soviet scientific establishment and thus had an insider's knowledge of Soviet methodology and a personal acquaintance with some of the longevity specialists. He also happened to come from a dissenter family. His father had been a purge victim, and he and his twin brother, Roy, a renowned scientist in his own right, were among the major liberal critics of the Soviet system, arguing for a more humanistic form of socialism. Shortly after he was forced into exile in the early 1970s, Zhores Medvedev was asked to comment on Soviet longevity claims. His views were published in *The Gerontologist* in October of 1974. In that article and in subsequent writings and interviews, he elaborated a number of scientific doubts about Soviet data and furnished political speculations on why they had been allowed to stand. His objections were manifold:[17]

> • Internal passports and other Soviet documents go back no further than 1932, at which time the original information was obtained through oral interviews, with no investigation made as to its authenticity. The census is taken the same way. Hence, in terms of verification, these records prove little.
> • No public official, church leader, or other person with a traceable career has been shown to be older than 108. Ages

have been highest where illiteracy is highest and records sparsest. Not one individual among the 500 claimed to be over 120 has pre-1932 documents.
• Soviet statistics have shown certain mathematical irregularities. For instance, in the 1959 census in the Altay region there were more people (19) in the 114–116 group than in the younger 111–113 group (14).
• Another odd finding in the 1959 census is that after age 100 male survivors begin to overtake females, and all claims of over 150 are male. This is contrary to the established worldwide pattern that longevous women outnumber longevous men in all age categories.
• Yet another statistical oddity from 1959 deals with survival through age 80. In Estonia, the region with the least longevity, out of each 100,000 persons born, 1,600 will survive to 80. In Georgia, the region with the second-highest longevity, that number will be 1,500. However, during the next twenty years, only 2 of the 1,600 Estonian octogenarians will survive to 100, compared with about 85 Georgians.
• Almost all settlements of any size in Georgia claim at least one centenarian, an improbable mathematical distribution.
• Physical and biochemical tests show results for some of the 100–110-year-olds that would be normal for persons not much older than 60. Similar tests on documented centenarians in other countries do not yield this result.
• Most Christian baptismal records were lost when 90 percent of the churches were destroyed between 1922 and 1940, yet Christians have a lower rate of centenarian claims than Moslems, who do not keep any birth records and may observe ten-month years. Older developed Christian cultures, like those in Armenia, have longevity rates similar to those in most European nations, even though Armenia is in the longevity belt of the Caucasus. Unlike many Moslem groups who rebelled against tsarist and Soviet policies, creating a need for some rebels to take new identities for safety and generally distorting family genealogies, the Armenians sought Soviet protection following genocidal massacres in Turkey.
• In the Altay region, asserted longevity is higher among native people than among the Europeans who live with them, even though the Europeans have better standards of living and better access to medical care.
• The statistical odds against the supercentenarian marriages claimed are astronomical, even if a claim is for a second

marriage contracted when both parties were already past 60.
Even marriages in which both parties are centenarians would
be extraordinarily rare.

To these objections Medvedev added a number of political interpretations, most of them involving Joseph Stalin. He
believed that after the end of World War II, local Georgian
officials seeking to flatter the Georgian-born dictator began to
publicize stories about longevity in their area. One old
chestnut that was revived dealt with a woman said to be 180
who had lived in the same Gori district that had given birth
to Stalin himself. Just as important as these personal touches,
longevity was advertised as another example of the superiority of the Soviet system. Whether he believed in the stories
or not, the aging Stalin certainly did nothing to discourage
them. Like many rulers before him, he seemed to enjoy the
idea that among his subjects were the longest-living people in
the world.

Whatever the original factual basis, tales of Soviet longevity soon got out of hand. Individuals, villages, and districts had always been zealous about making age claims.
Now, with the sanction of the state, older and older centenarians were "discovered." The phenomenon began to blend
with the wider question of Georgian uniqueness and desire
for greater autonomy. Within the Caucasus, regions like
Azerbaijan began to compete with Georgia, and within
Georgia ethnic minorities like the Abkhasians began to
compete with the Georgians. Soviet investigators exposed
claims that were off by whole decades, with individuals,
particularly men, doubling and even tripling their real ages.
One hoax involved a man living in Siberia who announced he
was 130. His photograph was published throughout the
U.S.S.R. and happened to be spotted by Ukrainian villagers
who recognized him as a man who had used his father's
papers to get out of military service in World War II. His real
age was 78. Although this and many other claims were

debunked by Soviet officials, Medvedev feels that many of the remaining claims are just as fraudulent.

Another element in Medvedev's political critique touched on the reliability of Soviet statistics. At the end of World War II, a report was released which stated that the average life-span in the U.S.S.R. had jumped from the low twenties to the high fifties. Given the invasion of the Nazis and the difficult times before, this was indeed a marvelous improvement. However, the Western press pointed out that the average life-span in the capitalist bloc had already reached into the high sixties. A short time later, revised Soviet statistics showed that the U.S.S.R. had caught up. The quick leap in the average life-span was then followed by a flat line for nearly a decade. Medvedev thought that by the 1970s the average life-spans in the developed world were about the same and that the flat line was a false correction needed to compensate for the false leap which had indicated parity before it had actually been achieved. Medvedev contended that other longevity data have been tampered with from similar political motives. He also noted that many statistics of totally unrelated kinds are still difficult to obtain. He cited such nonmilitary data as the number of high school pregnancies, the incidence of venereal disease, and the per capita consumption of alcohol.

Medvedev's skepticism did not lead him to conclude that there is no unusual longevity in the Caucasus, only that the claims are inflated. Among Soviet scientists he had spoken with confidentially before his exile, none had seen a person they believed to be older than 112. In that regard, Medvedev noted that the fabled Shirali Mislimov had not been accessible to foreigners, ostensibly either because he was too frail or because he was living in a security zone. The lack of an autopsy report after his death was equally suspicious.

Response to Medvedev's critique reflected his own blend of science and politics. Those who had been alienated by Soviet secrecy and bureaucracy found his views a con-

firmation of their own fears that the Soviets cannot be
trusted. As with everything else, these critics insisted that
outside verification was necessary before the longevity
claims could be accepted. In 1976, Dr. Jeffrey Bada, a 32-year-
old organic chemist at the Scripps Institute of Oceanography
in San Diego, directly challenged Soviet experts. He announced that his recently developed method for dating the
age of fossils through changes in their amino acid molecules
could be used to determine the age of humans. All that was
required was a tooth fragment from a living or recently
deceased centenarian. While the Soviets could perform the
procedure on their own, using his published work as a guide,
Bada volunteered to do the job personally in cooperation with
whatever scientists the Soviets designated. As of 1980, while
various delegations visiting the United States have expressed
interest in Bada's still controversial method, there has been
no official action.

Critics of Medvedev felt that his dredging up of the
Stalinist past was inappropriate at a time when Soviet science
and society were moving into a period of expanding liberty.
They thought his publications served the war hawks in each
political system better than they served the cause of science.
As for his specifics, they noted that Soviet scientists had been
reexamining and refining their work constantly, trying to
resolve issues of the very type troubling Medvedev. Naturally, there had been mistakes. The Thomas Parr myth still
took in the gullible. Why should the situation in the Soviet
Union be any different? And although inexperienced investigators, charming braggarts, and eager reporters had un-
doubtedly distorted Soviet surveys, the exposure of fraud had
been the work mainly of Soviet researchers and not of
outsiders. One also had to bear in mind that since supercentenarians did not exist elsewhere, established longevity patterns might not apply. Meanwhile, record keeping on all
levels had become more dependable, and the new census was
being planned with the greatest care ever, especially in regard
to centenarian claims.

The heat generated by Soviet findings came down to three essential issues: Were there really as many centenarians as claimed? Were they as vigorous as advertised? Were there hundreds of living supercentenarians? These questions could not be left in limbo the way an isolated claim like Anai Dollo's might, for they dealt on a massive scale with the fundamental question of the limits and nature of human longevity. But to assess all Soviet data, point by point and region by region, would require an effort approaching the massive scale of the original work. The author of this book concluded that a more reasonable and practicable approach would be to single out a particular geographical area for intensive firsthand observation with the orientation of an investigative reporter. The immediate objectives would be to examine Soviet research methods, to question officials on the doubts expressed about their data, to evaluate how longevity was presented to the Soviet public, and to meet with alleged centenarians. If the results of the investigation were conclusive, a generalization based on printed materials might be possible for Soviet research as a whole.

The choice for an on-site study was not difficult. The 1970 census had established Abkhasia, an autonomous region within Georgia, as the longevity capital of the world. Here, where the old were referred to as the "long-living," a population of half a million had produced no fewer than 294 centenarians, including 39 persons between 110 and 119, and 15 persons beyond 120. Among the supercentenarians was Shirali Mislimov's female counterpart, Khfaf Lazuria, "the oldest woman in the world," who had died in 1975 at the reputed age of 140. None of the centenarians lived more than 100 kilometers from the main highway, and the entire region, which is the size of Delaware, was open to foreign visitors. Films, articles, and books based on Abkhasia had appeared in the West for years, and the Abkhasian centenarian chorus was celebrated worldwide. Over half a dozen Americans had made longevity studies of some kind in Abkhasia between 1966 and 1977, providing a parallel American reference base to Soviet materials. All these factors made one more visit from the outside far less threatening than a request to see people in the restricted zones of Azerbaijan might have been. The journey was approved for the autumn of 1978. It was to result in a startling confirmation of both Soviet integrity and many of Medvedev's doubts.

2

THE LONG-LIVING PEOPLE
OF ABKHASIA

> A fat man on a horse is ridiculous.
>
> —*Abkhasian proverb*

The Caucasian mountain range straddles the border of the Soviet Union, Turkey, and Iran, linking the Black and Caspian seas. Its peaks, the highest in Europe, range over 18,000 feet above sea level. For centuries armies marching south from Moscow and Kiev battled forces coming northward from Teheran, Damascus, and Byzantium for control of vital passes. Legendary world conquerors such as Tamerlane, Genghis Khan, and Alexander the Great spread the fingers of their empires into its rugged valleys. Still earlier, poets sang of the exploits of Amazon warriors and how Prometheus, who dared to bring fire to the human race, was chained to a great rock in the same mountains where Noah's ark was said to have touched land, near the summit of Mt. Ararat. Here too came Jason in search of a real or proverbial golden fleece.

The strength and vigor of the people of the Caucasus are so striking that in the mid–eighteenth century Johann

Blumenbach chose their name to represent all people of European origin, and some decades later romantic poets like Pushkin and Lermontov renewed the fame of the "cradle of myth" throughout the continent. Cantankerous and rebellious subjects of whatever political rule they fell under, by the turn of the twentieth century the inhabitants of the Russian Caucasus were extremely displeased with the Romanov Dynasty. They would furnish some of the top leadership of the October Revolution.

Abkhasia, an autonomous area within the Georgian Republic and located at the western end of the Black Sea, is typical of the modern Caucasus. A sturdy, recently built two-lane highway hugs its 250 kilometers of coastline, with the southern end veering over the mountains to Tbilisi, capital of Georgia, and the northern continuing along the coastline to Sochi and other resort cities. At midpoint is Sukhumi, the area's administrative center. Founded as Diascuria by Greeks in the fifth century B.C., Sukhumi now has a population of a little over one hundred thousand, while Abkhasia as a whole has more than a half-million inhabitants, made up of some thirty ethnic groups. The largest is the Abkhasian nationality, which has its own language, culture, and history. Georgians are the second-largest group. There are also significant numbers of Armenians, Russians, Ukrainians, Greeks, and Turks, all of whom retain their separate identities. The three official languages of the area are Abkhasian, Georgian, and Russian, and many signposts and other government communications are in all three languages.

The person most qualified to speak of the realities of longevity in Abkhasia is Dr. Shoto Gogoghian, Director of the Institute of Gerontology, a local unit of the Academy of Medical Science. The institute, which has a staff of 3 medical doctors and 4 technicians, has quarters at present on the ground floor of a newly built but modest housing development a few kilometers beyond the central Sukhumi railroad station on the main route north. On one wall of its foyer there is a series of easy-to-read charts summarizing the major longevity findings of the past decade. Directly opposite is a photographic exhibit of the oldest Abkhasians.

The neat displays, of value to both expert and lay person, are characteristic of Gogoghian's outgoing and unassuming professional style. Before taking his present post in 1976, Gogoghian had been Director of Public Health in Abkhasia for twenty-three years, and his overall demeanor was much like that one would expect of any American counterpart. Whenever possible, his statements were precise; and when exactitude was not possible, his phrasing tended to be cautious rather than effusive. He was scrupulous about identifying some opinions as controversial or only a working hypothesis.[1]

The need to press possibly embarrassing challenges to centenarian claims was averted, as Gogoghian volunteered the view that probably no one in the world had ever attained 120 years of age and that most definitely no one in Abkhasia had. This disclaimer was a stunning departure from many previously published Soviet opinions. It was even more startling coming in Abkhasia, which had been widely proclaimed the mecca of superlongevity. When asked about the famous Khfaf Lazuria, Gogoghian replied that there was no doubt she had been an extremely old woman, perhaps the oldest in the history of the world, but Khfaf Lazuria had not been 140! Although admitting that some officials disagreed with him, Gogoghian thought Lazuria had not attained even 120 years of age. Questioned about the amino acid test developed by Bada, Gogoghian replied that it was known to him and other Soviet specialists. This was immediately followed by a reaffirmation that the conclusion that 120 was the outer boundary of achieved human longevity was based on numerous physiological examinations of centenarians, living and dead, and on familiarity with the longevity data available through frequent national conferences and consultations.

One doesn't have to be an accredited diplomat to know when a point should not be pursued further. If a tooth that could be proved to be more than 120 years old had been found, we can be certain it would have been displayed with the marvelous pomp and stagecraft the Soviets are noted for. Instead, Gogoghian stated that earlier age estimates had been exaggerated, often on hearsay or fragmentary evidence. There had been too many amateurs in the field, and as far as he was concerned, one of his major tasks was to ensure a scientific basis for future longevity studies. For him the objectives of the institute were fourfold: 1) discover how long the oldest Abkhasian had really lived; 2) determine the number of genuine centenarians; 3) identify the factors contributing to their long life; and 4) attempt to replicate the prolongevous factors for the benefit of the general population.

To meet his objectives, Gogoghian had set his team the task of visiting each of the 294 centenarians identified in the 1970 census. He personally had visited 178 of them and his colleagues had seen another 50, for a total of 228 contacts. Most of those not seen had died before they could be interviewed. Gogoghian explained that although the geographical area of Abkhasia was not large, roads to the villages were difficult to use most of the year, communications were still inadequate, and centenarians moved about unexpectedly or were sometimes too ill to hold long conversations or undergo arduous physical examinations. Field work was primarily limited to the summer months.

Gogoghian produced a tin box filled with the small white index cards familiar to researchers throughout the world. Each centenarian had a card, and in a nearby cabinet were corresponding files containing completed questionnaires and the results of various physical examinations. Gogoghian hoped that testing could be done annually to monitor the health of the long-living, but clearly one of his prime objectives was to make sure people aged only one year at a time. The institute also had begun tracking 200 nonagenarians in Sukhumi proper and the easier-to-reach hamlets. While he did not expect to see the final outcome of his work, Gogoghian expressed considerable pride that he had established a system which could resolve all future supercentenarian claims in Abkhasia.

The profile of Abkhasian longevity he outlined was compatible with findings elsewhere in the world. Earlier reports to the contrary notwithstanding, longevous women outnumbered longevous men by 2 to 1 in all age groups. Most of the centenarians (189) died shortly after their hundredth birthdays, with another large drop of 51 deaths occurring between 105 and 109. Putting another statistical nail into the supercentenarian coffin, Gogoghian reported that only a score or so of the 294 centenarians of 1970 were still alive. These included one supposed supercentenarian, Biga Vouba (123), whose claim Gogoghian considered definitely untrue, and another person of 116 whose age Gogoghian also doubted. Most of the long-living were rural people, often slightly built, who had lived arduous lives, particularly in their youth. Generally, they moved higher into the mountains during the summer months, and frequently men climbed to even higher areas to herd sheep or to hunt. Centenarians were spread among all the national groups. One hundred thirty-two were Abkhasians, 108 Georgians, 42 Armenians, 3 Greeks, 2 Russians, 2 Ukrainians, 2 Hebrews, 2 Turks, and 1 Azerbaijanian.

Half of the centenarians were able to function fairly well, taking care of major daily needs, while the other half required some degree of assistance. The most common disability was some hearing impairment. All lived with their families, and almost all had been married for the greater part of their lives, many having second or third spouses. In a study Gogoghian published in 1964,[2] 80 percent of all Abkhasians over 90 were described as mentally healthy and outgoing, a little over 45 percent had good hearing, and a little over a third had good vision. Only 10 percent were judged to have poor hearing, and fewer than 4 percent had poor eyesight. Evaluations of the health of men and women were comparable in all categories except the rather ominous "decrepit" ranking, which took in 18.2 percent of the women a opposed to only 8.7 percent of the men. In contrast, the "healthy" category included 35 percent of both sexes. One could surmise that the proud Abkhasian males were likely to conceal their failing health, while the Abkhasian females, trained in modesty, spoke more truthfully. In any case, the physical well-being of the longevous was remarkable, and the findings of 1964 had not been significantly altered by subsequent observations.

One common thread mentioned by those interviewed was that few had ever stopped working. Instead, as they grew older, they had eased their schedules, working 3 to 5 hours rather than 8 to 10 or shifting from doing the heaviest physical tasks to lighter ones. Although no one was required to work after 60, owing to the state pension system, Abkhasians enjoyed physical labor so much that they would have been as angry at being denied the right to work as they had once been angry when landlords forced them to work when they wanted some time to hunt or race their beloved horses.

Commenting on age verification, Gogoghian observed that it was far more difficult for women to lie than for men. If a woman had a son of 40, she could not claim to be 100, for during Gogoghian's twenty-three years as head of public health in Abkhasia the oldest recorded childbearing was at age 47, and in the entire Soviet Union the oldest observed birth was by a woman of 55. The world record was 57 years and 129 days.[3] Thus, any supercentenarian woman who claimed giving birth beyond those limits was a double wonder of the world: the longest-living human being and the oldest recorded mother. Men, on the other hand, could claim to have fathered children between 60 and 100. Visitors were reminded that storytelling was a fine Abkhasian art. Exaggerated accounts which added a few years at a time were not rare, especially in a society where immense honor accumulated with age. Being beneficiaries of a strict patriarchal society, men told most of the stories and liked to extol their sexual longevity. Adding to the difficulties was the fact that many persons did not really know exactly when they were born.

About the only factor Gogoghian omitted was that many

Abkhasians had never been enthusiastic about fighting for the central government and had done their best to avoid military duty by claiming to be too old. More specifically, throughout the nineteenth century the Abkhasians had periodically revolted against the tsarist regime. Violent incidents connected to the unsuccessful attempts provided ample reason for men to assume the identities of relatives. Relations between the Russians and the Abkhasians had been so foul that in the 1870s many Abkhasians chose to migrate to Turkey. By the time of the October Revolution, there were more ethnic Abkhasians in that land than in tsarist Russia, and some of the traditional distrust of Moscow became attached to the new Soviet system.

When the revolutionaries took control of Abkhasia in the 1920s, it was a backward region with an average life-span in the 20s and an illiteracy rate of over 98 percent. Malaria was so rampant along the coast that no one lived in the Sukhumi lowlands. Soviet power began to deal decisively with the health situation. Mosquitoes were eradicated, swamps drained, and eucalyptus trees planted to give the area a drier and more healthful ecological character. By the 1950s, public-health measures had advanced Sukhumi from a wasteland to a resort region. No less a personage than Joseph Stalin had a villa in the immediate vicinity, where he took advantage of the year-round warm weather. His example was followed by many dignitaries, including Lavrenti Beria, longtime head of the secret police. By the 1970s, Black Sea cruise ships accommodating Soviet and Eastern European tourists made regular dockings at Sukhumi, and Leonid Brezhnev had a retreat in nearby Pitsunda. In the lush hills overlooking the palm trees and subtropical vegetation of the coast were newly introduced crops grown on some of the nation's most successful collective farms. The average life-span had risen to 86 for women and 76 for men. Although the weight of 294 centenarians may have artificially elevated the averages. there could be no doubt that Soviet rule had given the formerly impoverished peasants unprecedented prosperity.

Throughout the talks with Gogoghian, concern for public health was emphasized. Much of the institute's work involved teaching Soviet health professionals how to care for the old and how to put into general practice what had been learned about health from the study of centenarians. As elsewhere in the U.S.S.R. and the developed world, the main killers in Sukhumi were heart disease and cancer. Trying to determine how centenarians had avoided these maladies was seen as a major practical as well as theoretical task. In attempting to address such longevity mysteries, Gogoghian had developed his own questionnaire, which he felt was superior to that used by other researchers.

Gogoghian pinpointed five factors contributing to Abkhasian longevity: respect for the aged, the nature of the life-style, the diet, the climate, and genetics. Of these, the reverence enjoyed by the old throughout the region is justly legendary. It is no exaggeration to say that this may be one of the few places in the world where people may genuinely look forward to old age. Traditional toasts include "May you live to be two hundred!" and "May you live to be as old as Moses [120]!" Even if an elder is ailing, his or her counsel is sought by all members of the family without a hint of any generational gap. Health permitting, the long-living preside over many official and informal social functions, enjoying numerous privileges. They are arbiters in family, village, and regional councils. For men, old age is the crown of a successful life; and for women, it is the only time when rough equality with men is finally possible. Many new freedoms accrue to women only after menopause. The psychological climate for the old is so positive that the rest homes available through government auspices are rarely utilized, as even in the smallest of families there are many relatives who covet the honor of housing an elder.

The Soviet authorities have incorporated this cultural phenomenon into their system by establishing a Soviet of Elders in each village to act as an advisory body to the formal government. When changes are being contemplated, the elders are among the first consulted. In the 1930s, some of them played leadership roles in the Collectivization campaigns by relating the new system to Abkhasian traditions of cooperative labor. Later, the long-living helped introduce new crops such as tea. During the war years and after, centenarians who continued to work were accorded honors as a part of drives to raise agricultural productivity. Often, too, elders are called upon to tell of the infamies and hardships of the tsarist era, and there is a holiday called the Day of the Long-Living People when they are feted.

Whatever their age, Abkhasians remain physically active. They follow regular and orderly daily patterns of hard work. Their routines have a tempo more linked to biological rhythms than the helter-skelter patterns that predominate in most developed nations. Abkhasians dislike being rushed, loathe deadlines, and never work to exhaustion. In the same vein, they consider it extremely impolite to eat quickly or to eat too much. Even after they pass the conventional age of retirement, they continue to work in the collectives and to walk many kilometers each day. Many chop wood, haul water, and bathe in mountain streams.

Cardiograms taken of Abkhasians show that some have suffered malfunctions or blockages of the type that would cause serious illness to sedentary people without feeling more than an upset stomach or experiencing a day of slight discomfort. Some studies of the cholesterol levels of centenarians have shown readings of 98 in a test in which the upper normal level for the middle-aged American would be 250. The cardiovascular benefits of their rigorous lives are enhanced during the summer when they move higher into the mountains. Although tobacco is grown in the area, few of the long-living people smoke.

The traditional diet followed by most of those who became centenarians contained between 1,500 and 2,000 calories a day. Seventy percent of that intake was from vegetables and dairy products. Fruits, nuts, grains, and a rare serving of meat made up the rest of the diet. (Many of the centenarians were nominal Moslems and had never eaten pork.) In addition, there was no coffee, tea, or sugar and little butter or salt. The major spice was red pepper, while honey was used as an occasional sweetener. A peculiarity of the diet not found anywhere else in Georgia was the avoidance of soups, a habit that seems to have no longevity significance. A further unique aspect of the traditional diet was the insistence on freshness. Vegetables were picked just before cooking or serving, and if meat was to be part of the menu, guests were shown the animal before it was slaughtered. Whatever the food served, all leftovers were discarded, because they were considered harmful to good health. Such concern for freshness guaranteed that a minimal loss of nutrients took place between garden and table. Most food was consumed raw or boiled, with nothing fried.

The combination of light eating and heavy exercise led to the lean somatype prized for both sexes. The Abkhasians have been among the few people in the world so appreciative of the ill effects of fat that even their children and infants remain slim. Moreover, the traditional Abkhasian body type was easy to maintain in the past, when considerable time was spent raising and training horses. From the earliest possible ages, even at 2 and 3, children were taught to ride. Horses provided the major sport, and the ability to do equestrian tricks was a mark of individual worth. The horses were never used as work animals, only for recreation and sports. For reasons not fully understood, despite their inferior social status, Abkhasian women participated in the horse culture in a manner unknown elsewhere in the Caucasus. They became accomplished riders and were so skilled in the martial arts that they played a fighting role in armed combat with enemies. Love of horses remains an Abkhasian passion, and horse parades are a favorite part of the Day of the Long-Living People celebrations.

The genetic influence on Abkhasian longevity was not much elaborated on by Gogoghian, who said that there was some speculation that certain blood types might be prolongevous and that longevous people usually claimed to have had longevous parents. It had been noted, however, that when people left the villages to go to cities or to other parts of the Soviet Union, their average life-spans tended to conform to those in the new territory, suggesting the primacy of environmental factors. There was less longevity in areas closer to industrialized coastal areas, where the terrain is flatter and where traditional customs have given way to many habits of the modern world.

Gogoghian's most controversial views involved climatic factors. Acknowledging that longevity had been observed in various climatic zones, he emphasized that Abkhasian centenarians lived the greater part of their lives at about 200 to 300 meters above sea level in a zone which experiences little snow or heavy winds. The mean temperature was 10 to 13 degrees Celsius, with minimal seasonal variations. Typically, homes were two-story dwellings in which only one room, the kitchen–dining area, was heated by a fireplace. To use Gogoghian's terminology, people in the villages are "slightly refrigerated." He believes this coolness serves to slow down the metabolism and may be a key factor in prolonging each stage of life.

Throughout his presentations, Gogoghian stressed that Abkhasian longevity research was still moving from a folkloric to a scientific basis, and visitors must be wary of their sources of information. This injunction proved to be well taken. In the United States, one would never accept the average newspaper story at face value or equate it with an article appearing in a scholarly journal. Nor would the views of the local chamber of commerce, tourist office, booster club, and politicians be accepted as gospel. The situation in the Soviet Union is no different, particularly in the Caucasus, where regional pride is intense. An investigator who treats the U.S.S.R. as a monolith and considers all government-linked information as "official" and therefore of equal weight will soon fall into error.

In Sukhumi, the sharpest contrast to Gogoghian's cautious views could be found in the Abkhasian State Museum.

While not included on the official Intourist tour of the city
for foreigners, the museum is visited extensively by Soviet
citizens.[4] The neat and well-laid-out premises devote part of
one room to a photographic display of centenarians and
nineteenth-century weapons, artifacts, and clothing. The
photos show 11 centenarians, of whom 8 are said to have
lived more than 132 years. Most are ethnic Abkhasians, but
there are immigrants like the Polish-born Yelif Kobachia
(105). Quite a few of these photos have been reproduced in
the Soviet press and are available to foreign publishers
through the Novosti News Agency. The distressing factor
about the photos is that the ages of the centenarians vary
tremendously from publication to publication—a subject to
be elaborated upon shortly. The personnel of the museum
who allowed photographs to be taken were genuinely convinced of the authenticity of the supercentenarians. They
were surprised by Gogoghian's opinions and stated that while
some exaggerations or doubts were possible, the essential
facts had been checked many times. Some of the supercentenarians had been locally famous for their musical or
handicraft skills and had verifiable histories. Like Gogoghian,
the museum officials were open with their material and
volunteered the names of centenarians, the villages where
they lived, and how to reach them through public transportation.

The museum director was in close contact with the
centenarian chorus, which is composed solely of men. Wearing national costume, the men sing traditional Abkhasian
songs and perform traditional dances at major celebrations.
Their luxuriant mustaches and high spirits have made them
beloved throughout the region. A booklet chronicling their
travels has been printed in Tbilisi, but as with so many Soviet
publications, demand for it so far exceeds the supply that
most officials do not even have a desk copy. At the Gerontological Institute, one of the inner corridors is decorated
with photographs clipped from the booklet. Some are candid

shots of major events, while others are posed in the villages to show typical scenes of bygone times.

To call the group a centenarian chorus, as is usually done, is to use a misnomer. The museum personnel stated that ever since the chorus was begun in the late 1930s, the minimum age has been 70, not the 100 a centenarian chorus would indicate or even the 90 told to many visitors. If the chorus really was limited to centenarians it would provide an impressive secondary verification for age claims, for it would mean that since the late 1930s Abkhasia has always had at least 20 centenarian men vigorous enough to sing and dance in public performances. Even if the minimal age were 90, such a chorus would be of some importance. With a starting age of 70, however, the main significance of the group is that it provides another illustration that older people not only can have a good time entertaining themselves but can also entertain and instruct others.

Another local Sukhumi institution where the maximal ages on longevity were favored was the local meeting hall, which also served as the chess and stamp club. Its walls were covered with dozens of photographs of national and international celebrities visiting Abkhasia. Many were shown in the company of centenarians. A picture of Ho Chi Minh sharing a toast at the Duripsh Collective is quickly pointed out to Americans. (This Soviet custom goes back to the 1920s, when the French author Henri Barbusse was toasted by Abkhasian supercentenarians.) Other photographs showed centenarians with Leonid Brezhnev and with Yuri Gagarin, the popular cosmonaut who made the first manned flight into space in 1961. Equally revealing of the role centenarians play in Abkhasian culture were photographs showing them posed with young people, publicizing productivity campaigns, in which the young were implored to emulate the hardworking elders. Discussions at the club as well as other interviews with Sukhumi residents revealed that the general population was convinced of Abkhasian longevity. Everyone had heard of at least one supercentenarian, although few had met any personally. Longevity stories usually elicited pride in the uniqueness of the Caucasus rather than any thought that it was linked to socialism.

What emerged as a semiofficial line on longevity was presented most ably by Riso Katchelavo, head of the Intourist Bureau at the Hotel Abkhasia. Katchelavo spoke a number of languages, including Georgian, Abkhasian, Russian, English, and two forms of Greek (Pontian and modern). He had traveled outside the Soviet Union and had often accompanied official guests doing field work among the centenarians. Without denying tourists the right to visit any Soviet citizen, he stated that the authorities felt it was best not to "bother" the long-living people unless there was an official delegation, of which fewer and fewer were thought desirable. There had been altogether too much publicity on the subject, and the government felt its centenarians were being exploited and that supercentenarians were an endangered species. His own private opinion was that Abkhasian longevity had entered a new stage. With the increasingly higher standard of living, there would be a paradox: the average life-span would increase and the percentage of centenarians decrease. This would happen because longevity seemed to be linked to arduous life-styles and restricted diets of a kind that were incompatible with the modern Soviet ethic. No one was going to walk 20 kilometers from Atara to Sukhumi when he or she could ride in a car or bus, and increasingly, people were enjoying more meat, pastries, coffee, butter, tea, and other antilongevous foods that had once been rare or totally unavailable.

This scenario blended nicely with Gogoghian's information that most of the 1970 centenarians had perished already. Inevitably this meant there could be only a handful of possible supercentenarians in the 1980 census, and perhaps none. Katchelavo's views would gracefully interpret the decline not as a health retrogression but as a function of progress. Left behind would be the legend that once upon a time in the land of the Amazons and Prometheus, there had been generations of supercentenarians.

Alas, the claims for supercentenarianism cannot be allowed to disappear so nimbly. If even one were valid, we would have to know everything about so important a life. The most promising candidate for investigation was Khfaf Lazuria, dubbed by one American journalist the "Coquette of the Caucasus." Renowned for her sense of humor, Lazuria loved to mug for the camera and had given countless interviews describing her long life. A tiny wisp of a woman at only 4 feet 2 inches, she had lived so long that she was treated "like a man." Her claim of 140 years at her death in 1975 would mean she had been born in 1835, during the reign of Tsar Nicholas I and the presidency of Andrew Jackson. Could it be true?

Alexander Leaf didn't think so. When he visited her in 1972, she was already claiming to be in her 141st year (b. 1832?). She told him she had been an inhabitant of her village all her life, contracting her first marriage at 16. Her first born son and her first husband were soon lost in a typhus epidemic. At 50 years of age, she married Lazuria and gave birth to another son, who was a grown man of 30 at the time of the Great Snow of 1910, when 2 meters fell in one night. That same year she took up smoking for the first time, and she had continued the habit at the rate of a pack a day ever since. She stated that both of her parents and one husband had passed the century mark. Judging one "big war in the North" to be the Crimean War of 1853–56 and another story to be linked to the Turkish Wars of 1873–78, the cautious Leaf concluded, ". . . I have arrived at a degree of confidence that prompts me to place Mrs. Lazuria's age close to 130. In the absence of written records this is my best estimate, and it should be regarded as only that—an unverifiable estimate."[5]

Two years later, Sula Benet heard a different story.[6] Now, Lazuria was officially 139 by virtue of register number 439 of the village, which showed a birthdate of October 18, 1835. To the longevous parents and spouse, Lazuria added one great grandfather who had lived to be 160 (one of whose grandsons lived to be 120) and a first cousin of 146. Instead of having been a lifelong resident of Kutol, she reported that she had been abducted by the Turks in 1853 while still a girl and not allowed to return home for ten years. There were four instead of two marriages. The one in which the husband and son are lost occurs at age 40 instead of 16. The marriage to Lazuria, for which she converted from Islam to Christianity, takes place around age 50 but with no children mentioned. Much more is said about her work in organizing collective farms and how she was a champion tea picker when already a centenarian. Tarkuk, the son of the Great Snow of 1910 story, is now identified in the village record as a stepson. After getting to know the family, Benet concluded the old woman smoked only when photographers were around, because she thought it made her look modern and jaunty. Before actually meeting Lazuria, Benet had been given information and photographs in 1972 in which Lazuria was identified as being 131 (b. 1841?).[7] A brother and 3 sisters were said to have lived to be about 90.

Neither the Leaf nor the Benet accounts match one given to Peter Young of *Life* in 1966.[8] At that time, Lazuria claimed to be 124 (b. 1842?). She admitted not knowing her exact birth date but said her parents had told her when she was 15 and she had kept track ever since. In this variation she states she was married to Lazuria at 50 and that Tarkuk was already 3 at the time.

Yet another version of her life was told to journalist Henry Gris in 1973.[9] At first Lazuria tried to claim to be 160 (b. 1813?), but she was restrained by relatives, who said she was only teasing and that her real age was 139 (b. 1835). Centenarianism was now accorded to the brother and 3 sisters, but instead of being kidnapped by Turks she had only heard stories about others who were. The abductions took place during the Makhadzhir Raids dating to a period between the Crimean War and Turkish Wars identified by Leaf. Instead of the four Benet marriages, there again were only two, but the first is not at 16 (as told to Leaf) but at 25. Lazuria is wed at age 48, and the birth of Tarkuk (the stepson of the Benet-Young accounts) takes place at age 53. She confides that she has been smoking cigarettes for a hundred years. When Gris asked how she could manage that in a culture where only widows and old women may smoke, Lazuria breezily assured him she knew where to hide.

Before joining the staff of the sensationalist *National Enquirer*, Gris had spent thirty years as a reporter for United Press International. Both jobs gave him practice in spotting tall tales. While appreciative of Lazuria's charm, he notes how Tarkuk made a discreet exit, to return some time later mounted on a horse and garbed in the traditional turban and cherkesska (Cossack uniform). He is aware too how the interpreter, a local poet, is "swollen with pride as though he were personally responsible for all centenarians encountered during the journey."[10] The same man will inform him that visitors to the grand old lady are expected to leave a small gift. In Gris's case it is a pencil flashlight, which is much appreciated. Enjoying the drinks, stories, and equestrian show, Gris begins to think of Khfaf Lazuria as a kind of Abkhasian superstar. She and her family had been through this routine countless times, and they tried their best to tell guests whatever they thought guests most wanted to hear. His comment upon her death in 1975 sums it up well: "Her life was, indeed, a great performance."[11]

Without straying from the "facts" provided by Leaf, Benet, Young, and Gris, the formula for Lazuria's supercentenarianism is obvious. Start with a generous serving of pride, exaggeration, playfulness, and gullibility. Mix in an illiterate's bowl where there are few documents predating the 1930s. Spice with "battles in the North" which might be feuds, raids, revolts, or wars spanning a fifty-year period which she may have been told about rather than have experienced. Drop in a son born after her 45th birthday who most probably is a stepson. Spike with from two to four marriages. Salt with the champion longevity family of all time, which includes centenarian grandparents, parents, brothers, sisters, husbands, and cousins. Pepper with a smoking habit that begins in 1874 or 1910 or after the Great Patriotic War, when she was definitely free enough to behave as a man. The concoction is pretty unstable, and Gogoghian, privy to even more information, had drawn the right conclusion. And if the superstar of longevity is a fraud, what about the other 293 centenarians?

Inconsistency of age claims is the rule. The same photograph of Solomon Arshba identifying him as 140 in the state museum was released to Benet with an age of 127.[12] A Novosti source advertised Alexa Tsvijba as 125, but Dr. Sichinava of Sukhumi consulted the most conventional identification and found him to be only 95.[13] Tandal Dzoupha of Chlou told visiting Americans in 1978 that he was 114.[14] Two years earlier he had been identified to the Dannon people as 97,[15] while three years before that he had told Leaf he was 102[16] and Gris that he was 104.[17]. In 1975, Benet reported that Kurt Zantariya had been verified by authorities as 119 in 1963,[18] yet in 1966 he was still only 120 for Peter Young. The *Life* journalist was told that Makhtil Targil of Duripsh was 102; but during the early 1970s Targil was still only 104 for Benet[19] and Leaf,[20] even though he managed 109 for Gris[21] and made a whopping 118 for the Dannon people in 1976. Sheilach Butba was identified to Benet as 111 in 1972,[22] but one year later his son informed Gris[23] that Sheilach was 128. That same year he went down to 120 for Leaf,[24] who judged him to be no more than 113. His wife's age zigzagged with her husband's, but the higher his stated age, the more the distance between them grew. Connected to Butba's claim was that of Kamachich Kvichenya, 137 years of age for her 1976 Dannon portrait, who told Gris she knew she was exactly two years older than Sheilach because when they were children the other girls had teased her by chanting, "Look at her, she loves Sheilach! And she's two years older!"[25] Kamachich, in turn, said she was only a shade younger than Khfaf Lazuria.

This list could easily be tripled without inclusion of factors like ages depending on doubtful facts. Cynics could draw the conclusion that every age claim is inflated and that there are no genuine centenarians. This would probably be as wrong as accepting the superlongevous claims at face value, for the secondary proofs and visible generations indicate advanced ages. Noticeable, too, is that the shakiest accounts are those by individuals trying to be over 115, while those hovering around 100 have much more internal consistency and more believable particulars.

Nor should the necessity of zeroing in on the ages detract from the amazing vigor of the long-living. Tandal Dzoupha, for instance, probably at least a nonagenarian, is an avid dancer and singer, his straight back and tall, elegant bearing immediately visible in photographs of the chorus. At 70, he would be a man to envy. Widower Makhtil Targil, the dean of the Duripsh centenarians, informed Sula Benet that he was seriously looking for a new spouse, and Kamachich Kvichenya kidded Gris about getting her a new American husband. Temur Tarba, who turned 100 in 1973, was still riding horses and had gotten a Hero of Labor award for cultivating corn while in his 90s. Their liveliness is typical of the long-living people throughout the region. The men like to dress up in the old uniforms, preside at banquets, and tell stories. The women, while less dramatic, are just as engaging and often quite candid in their remarks. Taking quality of life as a standard, there is considerable centenarian gold among the supercentenarian pyrite.

The historical record which intrigued Metchnikoff and Pavlov also is reassuring. Travel journals, literary works, and histories going back centuries refer to Caucasian longevity. A typical nineteenth-century traveler whose major interest was the brigandage and feuding then associated with the area offhandedly wrote of meeting a 120-year-old Armenian monk.[26] The man was described as sleeping most of the time as well as being blind and halt. One doesn't have to accept the claim to appreciate that advanced age was not considered remarkable. While few writers took a specific interest in longevity, asides about old people and observations about the honors accorded to village elders are constantly encountered in writing about the Caucasus. One pre–Soviet era traveler who was specifically interested in the long-living was Essed Bey, a man of Daghestani ancestry born in the city of Baku. In 1916, against the wishes of a father concerned for his safety, Bey took an extended horseback tour of the region. He concluded that once having reached adulthood, "The Caucasian, on the average, will attain the age of 80 to 90 years. Centenarians and even older persons are by no means uncommon."[27]

Evidence of a similar nature is found in the literary traditions of the ethnic Abkhasians. When the Soviets took power, fewer than 2 percent of the Abkhasians were literate in any language, and there was no alphabet for their spoken language. Three attempts to form an alphabet, mainly using Russian and Georgian characters, failed before the present system was adopted in 1954. Since that time, oral traditions going back to the ancient Nart epics have been written down, as have more recently composed songs and stories.[28] Longevity and the role of benevolent elders in society are frequent themes. Of particular note is that jokes and tall tales are favored forms of expression. One story repeated in many variations involves a centenarian being interviewed by an awed traveler (in the modern version: a gerontologist). The centenarian solemnly declares that the secret of long life is to avoid all alcohol and tobacco and to control one's temper. Suddenly, he is drowned out by shouting in the adjoining room. "Don't let that bother you," the poker-faced centenarian says. "That's just my older brother and my father. They've had too much to drink again and are having their usual argument over cigarettes and women."

The Abkhasian scholars who gather these stories often serve as assistants to longevity researchers. Unfortunately, the proofs of old age they innocently accept take in every error warned against by Thoms and Young. The repetition of hearsay and superficial evidence related by congenial old folks also has passed into the work of Sula Benet, the only American to write extensively about Abkhasia. While excellent in its cultural and historical descriptions, her work, which draws heavily on Soviet sources, leaves much to be desired in the area of age verification and reflects the gossipy nature of so much that is written about the Caucasus in the U.S.S.R. and abroad. Benet has an appallingly cavalier attitude toward the supercentenarian claims, writing, "It seems to be mere quibbling to discredit reports of longevity by questions about precise ages. If a person lives to 120 rather than 130 in health and vigor, the fact of old age is barely diminished."[29]

The mistakes that flow from such an outlook are evidenced in a story Benet tells about the 180-year-old woman from Gori referred to earlier. Giving no citations for her account, Benet reports that Metchnikoff interviewed the woman in 1904 and leaves the strong impression that he accepted the claim.[30] Metchnikoff's summation which appears in his *The Prolongation of Life* (1910) is quite different.[31] He refers to a newspaper clipping from the *Tiflissky Listok* of October 8, 1904, that has been sent to him by a kindly stranger. The news story tells of Thense Abalava, an Osete woman, living in the village of Sva, Gori district. It is not clear whether the newspaper reporter has investigated the claim personally or is relaying the tale at second or third hand. We must also note that although Metchnikoff was justifiably honored as a great scientist, he was no expert on age verification, accepting already disproved claims such as those of Thomas Parr and Drakenberg the Dane.

A similar retelling of a story by Benet touches on an episode from a history written by O. G. Butkov.[32] In 1722 and again in 1796, the rebellious city of Derbent had to be subdued by the Russians. In each instance, a delegation of elders presented the victors with a plate upon which lay a silver key to the city. On the second occasion, when the chief elder was asked to identify himself, he responded that he had already given his name seventy-four years earlier when he surrendered the city to the army of Peter the Great. He was now 120! A nice story, to be sure, but no documentation is offered to show that it is not a fable. Nor is it explained why the elders of 1722 were led by a man then only 46 years of age. Many stories of this nature, especially those told by centenarians, are passed along without critical comment or examination.

Benet presents a linguistic proof that is far more persuasive of Abkhasian longevity. In her 1976 book *How to Live to Be 100*, she writes that the people in the Caucasus, ". . . have specific terms or expressions for great grandparents going back to six generations. These expressions are used to refer to the living, not to those who have died. Very few languages contain expressions for so many generations of living relatives."[33] Her early study *The Abkhasians* (1974) was somewhat more conservative: ". . . the abundance of familiar names for such relatives as great-great grandfather is an indication that sufficient members of fifth-generational families exist to require their use."[34] In either case, the need for words to describe living relatives of fifth and sixth generations indicates a significant incidence of old age and probable longevity.

Other linguistic clues about longevity are less conclusive. For instance, Benet points out that Abkhasian language forms indicate the age relationship between speakers, so that there is a constant reaffirmation of who is younger and who is older. But all this means is that the relationships remain constant, not that the ages are correct. Thus Sheilach Butba acknowledges being younger than Kamachich Kvichenya, and Kamachich Kvichenya acknowledges being younger than Khfaf Lazuria. If Lazuria's age is posited as 120, Kvichenya drops to 118 from her high of 137, and Butba is no more than 116. If we accept Leaf's highest estimate that Butba is 113, Kvichenya drops to 115 and Lazuria to about 117—a considerable fall from her official 140. The same process would apply in Duripsh, where Makhtil Targil's age is the standard. In all these instances, ages given by the centenarians have varied considerably from year to year, with families, some authorities, and friends supporting the fluctuations.

Another argument favored by Benet is that the privileges of old age are so great that the genuinely longevous zealously guard their prerogatives against pretenders. This argument does not take into account the rivalry between villages, ethnic groups, and republics for having the oldest of the old. The view is further rebuffed by Benet's own observation that men will lie *downward*, claiming to be octogenarians when they are much older because a man of about 100 is thought to be in sexual decline. Sexuality in general is a whirlpool of longevity exaggerations, as can be seen in numerous claims of women who give birth after 55 and men who become fathers after 90. A reasonable conclusion could be drawn that the astounding virility among the old and the longevous belongs to the same class of lore as the Thomas Parr stories. Then too, peasants traditionally have enjoyed pulling the legs of their city cousins, and as their literature illustrates, the Abkhasians' sense of humor is hardly underdeveloped. The difference between 92, 102, and 122 may not be taken quite as seriously by peasants as by gerontologists. Since everyone in the village knows the truth anyway, what's the harm in having some fun with the outsiders? By Benet's own admission, even she thinks the difference between 120 and 130 amounts to "mere quibbling." We can assume that some of her Soviet colleagues share her view. They are not all as meticulous as Shoto Gogoghian.

The final authorities to consult in these matters are, of course, the centenarians themselves. One person whose claim of 110 was considered legitimate by Sula Benet, Shoto Gogoghian, and the museum director was Vanacha Temur of Lichny, a man often spoken of as among the healthiest and more vigorous of the centenarians. Without making any preannouncement of intent or seeking official aid, a group of investigators made a trip to the farm where Vanacha Temur has lived all of his long life. The first measure of the old man's authority was that his son would not open the garden gate until he secured his father's approval for the visit.

Wearing a snappy leather hat, the venerable, always referred to only by his first name, walked smartly across the garden and took up the responsibilities of a host. Spotting an infant among his guests, Vanacha insisted that a cow be milked so that the baby could have some wholesome country refreshment. For the other guests baskets of apples from his best tree and a round of drinks were brought out. Only when these essentials were accomplished was he prepared to speak.

Familiar with international protocol, Vanacha talked of the need for world peace and increased understanding among nations before proceeding to speak about himself. Unlike most of the other centenarians, he had a baptismal certificate. According to the dates of this document, he was 106, but he explained that his baptism had been delayed until he was in his fourth year because his parents lacked funds to pay the priests. Although this was an echo of an excuse Thoms had frequently encountered, Vanacha's vigor, even at 106, was incredible. A man of about five feet with twinkling blue eyes and an elegant white mustache, he was the personification of a kindly and playful grandfather. He credited his slim, wiry body to light eating, horseback riding, farming, and walking in the mountains. These days he slept more than he used to, but he felt fine and was looking forward to the sixty-first anniversary of the Revolution, for the chorus was going to be filmed beside the ten-centuries-old Basletsky Bridge near Sukhumi for a program to be shown on national television.

The chorus was obviously one of Vanacha's great joys. He loved being with the other old men and being fussed over. In photographs of the group his impish antics were frequently the focus of attention. He said that he had helped form the group forty years earlier. At that time, he was 70 and one of the youngest members; now he was the oldest continuous member and probably the chorus elder. Again, the round numbers were somewhat suspicious, but it is unlikely that he was less than 65 at the time of the chorus's establishment, which would indicate the same general age as the baptismal record. Asked if the chorus would like to perform in the United States, Vanacha thought it would be a lot of fun, but that it wouldn't happen because a lot of them, himself included, did not like to fly. They wouldn't even take a plane to Moscow. So perhaps it would be better if the Americans came to Abkhasia. He obligingly clipped on an "I Love New York" button as a gesture of camaraderie.

After more than an hour's conversation, there was a round of toasting. Vanacha drank two full tumblers of a strong applejack and confirmed that many of the long-living liked to take one shot every morning to get going. Otherwise, they drank only on festive occasions. He brought the interview to a close by embracing each of his visitors, lingering longest over the infant now sated with fresh milk. As he walked back to his house, he looked like a man who would be around to greet visitors for many years to come. The laurel of Abkhasian longevity clearly had passed into his hands, and Vanacha Temur was handling it with the same dignity and joy as Khfaf Lazuria once had.

A centenarian with a contrasting personality was Mikhail Kaslantzia. The chorus did not interest him, and except for one time when a Japanese television crew had posed him with his neighbor Khfaf Lazuria, he had not participated in the centenarian boom. He was like Pierre Joubert in that age did not concern him. "I'm pretty sure I'm over a hundred. I was fifty when I married my wife, who was then seventeen. Now she is seventy, so I must be about a hundred and three. It isn't important." Always speaking in Abkhasian, he expressed interest in seeing photographs of other longevous people. Without using glasses, he studied the hands of an Ecuadorian peasant woman. "These are beautiful hands. They have done work," he said. Then, when he spotted a full-page color photo of Khfaf, his whole manner changed. He chortled and called his wife to his side for a good look.

Khfaf's photograph set Mikhail to telling stories of how he, Khfaf, and others had begun the first tea collectives. They had all been champion tea pickers, he said, and striking a chord generally left untouched by others, he announced with considerable relish that he had joined the Communist Party in 1919 before the Revolution took power in Abkhasia. He had been part of the local political bureau, and with energetic hand motions he described the gun battles fought with local landlords. As far as he was concerned, the only good thing about life before the Revolution had been the trips into the mountains he made as a young man when he had the time to walk and hunt all summer. Up there he had been so free that he felt that if he wanted to fly all he had to do was spread out his arms. He spoke, too, of how he liked to eat the grasses of Abkhasia, by which he meant various leafy greens that grew wild and were the favorites of the older generation. "We didn't eat so much in the old days. Life was difficult."

An unusual feature of the small but immaculate Kaslantzia home was that even though it was the middle of a weekday afternoon, the center table was filled with snacks and drinks as if many guests were anticipated. Mikhail's wife quietly explained that their only child, an adopted son, had died four years before in an automobile accident. As a memorial, they had vowed to leave the table set just as it had been that night. Outside, a very large portrait of a handsome young man in his 30s could be seen attached on one wall of the house. The accident, which destroyed the continuity of generations, had obviously taken much out of their lives, but the Kaslantzias did not allow their grief and mourning to make them unduly somber. Like Vanacha, they scolded their guests for not having announced the visit beforehand. Next time, they wanted to prepare a proper Abkhasian feast, and the Americans were not allowed to leave before promising there would indeed be a next time.

Anyone who cares to roam the Abkhasian hinterland will soon discover that in the courtyards of the neatly kept homes there will invariably be older persons identified as being at least in their 80s. Other older people can be encountered walking up and down steep roads or chatting at rural bus stops. Contact with them, like contact with centenarians such as Vanacha and Mikhail, illuminates the special magic of old age in Abkhasia. These are not cardboard role models from a propaganda offensive, but very real, very winning people with a full complement of individual idiosyncrasies. Generally, they look forward to reaching 100 and give every indication of a genuine contentment with their lives. With little prodding, they will talk about food, horses, family life, or whatever else interests the visitors. Their symbolic and real leadership in social and family affairs dramatizes the foolishness of the notion that life after 65 needs to be bleak and unrewarding.

From a strictly statistical standpoint, the final count on Abkhasian longevity must wait until the dashes following the birth dates are finally recorded on all the index cards kept for the 1970 nonagenarians and centenarians at the Gerontological Institute. Yet even now the main contours of Abkhasian longevity have been established. This is a region where longevity has been celebrated in stories, jokes, and songs for hundreds of years. From the first attempts at scientific verification made at the turn of the century through the centenarian fad of the 1970s, the peasants have amused themselves by inflating their ages. If the popular press, nationalist elements, and ambitious politicans have sometimes gone overboard with the centenarian hoopla, then just as clearly the gerontologists have tried their best to pull on the reins to give a more scientific appraisal.

The frequency of exaggeration should not obscure the likelihood that extraordinary longevity exists. If the 1970 census is accurate, Abkhasia would have a longevity rate 20 times that of the United States. But even if as many as 90 percent of the claims were false, the percentage would still be significant, and most of the fakers would be remarkable nonagenarians. The recent history of Abkhasia shows that as traditional infectious diseases have been tamed by public-

health measures, the major modern killers, heart diseases and
cancers, are inhibited by indigenous traditions. Factors such
as the nature of the traditional diet, strenuous physical
activity throughout life, the hilly terrain, rhythmic patterns
of work, a pollution-free environment, and the unique psychological support enjoyed by the long-living figure heavily
in the longevity phenomenon. It is also likely that someone
in the region has lived longer than Delina Filkins, but much
more detailed proofs would have to be provided before any
prudent investigator could accept any of the official ages as
truly verified, and the chance that anyone has lived to over
120 is extremely unlikely.

As more and more people throughout the world begin to
achieve their 80s and 90s, Abkhasia will be even more
important as an illustration of how fully the sunset years can
be enjoyed. The final images of this rugged land truly belong
to the elders: To women like Khfaf Lazuria threading a needle
without benefit of glasses and to men like Vanacha Temur
doing a fancy step for their friends. To couples like Makhtil
and Dzyrkuy Khagva proudly posed before the beautiful
walnut house the husband constructed for them long ago. To
Makhtil Targil taking a daily bath in a cold mountain stream;
to Kamachich Kvichenya giving toasts alongside the men; to
Teb Sharmat explaining a traditional instrument to a
Sukhumi scholar; to Rahiama Butba feeding her prize flock of
black turkeys; to Temur Tarba galloping his favorite horse.
Such elders are never referred to as the old but always as the
long-living. The Russian word for them is *dolgozhiteli*.

3

SOVIET CENTENARIANS

> We will be quite satisfied if we
> manage to reverse the process of
> premature aging and sustain the bio-
> logical age commensurate with the
> calendar age; thus assuring man a
> life span of well over a hundred
> years.
>
> —Dimitri Chebotarev

The heartland of Soviet longevity is composed of the three
Caucasian republics: Azerbaijan, Georgia, and Armenia. Together they account for over 25 percent of the nation's 19,000
centenarians, but most gerontological interest has been
focused on Georgia, where the study of centenarianism has
gone on for the longest period and where the level of research
has the highest sophistication. This is in contrast to the
flamboyant claims characteristic of Azerbaijan and the
lower-keyed approach favored in Armenia. The 1970 census
showed 1,844 centenarians (including the 294 Abkhasians) in
the total Georgian population of about 5 million. This works
out to 39.3 centenarians per 100,000 of population. The
Azerbaijan figures work out to 48.2 centenarians per 100,000
and the Armenian to 24.3 per 100,000. In most developed
nations there are from 3 to 5 centenarians per 100,000 of
population.[1]

Any uniqueness in Soviet longevity falls or stands on the situation in the Caucasus, but Soviet gerontology has hardly been limited to that area. Probably no other modern state has devoted as much energy to longevity research over so long a period. The scale of the Soviet effort can be appreciated by a look at the massive project undertaken in the 1960s by the Gerontological Institute of Kiev.[2] Working from the 1959 census, the project involved the questioning of 40,000 persons over 80 years of age, with a physical examination given to 27,181 participants. The findings were strikingly similar to those of work done in other nations with much smaller groups of people and were similar to the findings in Abkhasia.

The Kiev project discovered that the overwhelming majority of those Soviet citizens over 80 had been employed as either farm workers or manual laborers. Fewer than 4 percent were teachers, office workers, medical workers, and the like. A high percentage had worked at the same occupation all their lives, including a resounding 90 percent of the manual workers. As in Abkhasia, most were found to have lean bodies and to be moderate eaters. Ninety-one percent reported they ate a mixed diet, 8.4 percent a vegetarian diet, and .6 percent a meat-oriented diet. The state of their health at the time of the survey was quite good. Seventy percent did all their own household chores, and 55.4 percent moved about unaided. Forty-four percent of the men and 31 percent of the women were judged to be practically healthy, which was defined to mean that their lives were no more affected by illness or disease than were the lives of those in younger age brackets. Ninety-seven and one-half percent of the women and 45 percent of the men had never smoked. Of possible sociopsychological importance, 99 percent of the men and 97 percent of the women had been married at least once.

The organizer of this study was Dr. Dimitri Fedorovich Chebotarev (sometimes spelled Chebotaryov), the director of the Institute, a member of the Academy of Medical Science, and the leading Soviet authority on longevity. Drawing from the intimate knowledge of all Soviet gerontological research, by the 1970s Chebotarev had observed five prolongevous constants:[3]

1. The longevous tend to work continually throughout their lives. As they grow older, the volume of work diminishes but the longevous never totally retire. Their work and their lives follow rhythmical patterns so that energy is expended over a period of time in regular quantities rather than in short or spasmodic bursts of frantic energy broken by rest periods or carried to exhaustion. The work of the longevous is physically demanding.
2. The longevous abstain from rich foods which can cause overweight and its associated health problems. Their diets are low in fat, sugar, and salt while being high in vitamins. Their cholesterol levels are low. The daily caloric intake is usually less than 2,000. While alcoholic drinks are usually part of the diet, consumption is moderate.
3. The longevous tend to do the same kind of work throughout life with the longest living often remaining in the same village or region as their parents and relatives. Many live in mountain areas and when older people move to cities or away from their immediate families, their death rate is high.
4. The longevous are most highly concentrated where "local tradition demands respect for elders."
5. The longevous report having long-living relatives suggesting genetic influence of some kind, although the specific role of heredity has not been clearly determined.

One notable divergence from the observations made by Gogoghian in Abkhasia is that Chebotarev had eliminated climatic conditions as a major factor. He also eliminated other locally based theories, such as the idea that the nature of cosmic radiation at the altitudes where most of the longevous people in the Caucasus are found may be of importance. Looking at the long-living phenomenon from a broad national perspective, Chebotarev had discounted such influences as being geographical idiosyncrasies rather than longevity universals.

Similarly, while Chebotarev included possible genetic factors in his top five, other commentary indicates this to be lip service to an undeniable influence rather than a strong conviction of its centrality. A possible explanation for this attitude may be that in the 1960s study there was a surprisingly low incidence of immediate blood relatives over 80 years of age.[4] The high of 40 percent was reached in the Ukraine, where longevity is not particularly pronounced, while in Abkhasia the rate was an unexpectedly low 31 percent. With so many of the longevous people living in the same region, even in the same village or household, as their parents, the similarity in environment and life-styles could account for such a percentage quite as satisfactorily as genetics.

That the deemphasis on genetics is more than a holdover from the period when the subject was a Soviet taboo is supported by studies made in the United States. Contrary to the old aphorism that the best way to be longevous is to have longevous parents, various investigations indicate that having longevous parents adds only an average of three years to the life-span.[5] While not a totally insignificant factor, this advantage can be compared to the five years that are gained by simply living in the country or the eight years that are lost by smoking one pack of cigarettes a day. This consensus in American and Soviet research casts additional doubt on the frequent assertions by supercentenarians that both of their parents and many close relatives also were longevous.

Soviet studies are usually most reliable when they deal with objective data and identify longevity factors found in mammoth samplings. In the area of age verification of specific individuals they are far weaker, with numerous indications of wishful thinking or sloppy methodology. Little commentary, for example, can be found on the limited number of generational offspring from presumed centenarians. Simple arithmetic shows that if one starts with a newborn infant (one generation), one can derive a mother of 18 (two generations), a grandmother of 36 (three), a great grandmother of 54 (four), a great-great grandmother of 72 (five), and a great-great-great grandmother of 90 (six). Just such a family is documented in Dorothy Gallagher's *Hannah's Daughters—Six Generations of an American Family: 1876–1976.* Oral histories, genealogical charts, and photographs establish the identity of each member of the family. Included is a photograph showing Hannah (97), the family elder, holding Susan (2), the family baby.[6] The work, it should be noted, is not directed toward longevity concerns but sought to document the ways in which the lives of women have changed over a hundred-year period.

Gallagher's family was not unique. In the 1890s, Alexander Graham Bell, the inventor of the telephone, had become interested in families with a history of long life.[7] One remarkable clan was that mothered by Lavinia McMurray. She had four generations of offspring, 107 living descendants, by the time she was 85. Birth records were available for the family, and each member was clearly identifiable in four group photographs of the five generations together. McMurray's son Robert and her daughter Mrs. J. B. Gregory also parented four generations of offspring. If Lavinia had lived to be a centenarian, she would have had five generations of offspring at age 105 traceable through either her daughter or her son. Bell located another family headed by Mrs. Karl Medlen, age 89. Her daughter was 61, her granddaughter 41, her great granddaughter 21, and her great-great granddaughter 7 months. If this pattern of motherhood at about age 20 had continued, a sixth generation would have been achieved when Mrs. Medlen was 109.

Bell's 4 five-generational families in which the eldest was not even longevous does not mean that other four- or five-generational families might not include centenarians— simply that they cannot be thought of as giving it proof. The Gallagher example of a six-generation family with the eldest being less than 100 demonstrates that only a seven-generation family would be a strong indication of supercentenarianism. If, as is claimed in the Soviet Union, there are many thousands of centenarians, there should be a considerable number of six-generational families and perhaps some of seven generations. But this is not the case.

The explanation most often advanced, that they married late in life, is contradicted by many individual histories. Typical in this respect is Shirali Mislimov, who first married in his 20s. A broader analysis of age at marriage in the Caucasus was made by Sula Benet, who determined that the usual age of marriage for Abkhasian women in modern times is an unremarkable 20–23[8] and that marriages in Azerbaijan occur at earlier ages.[9] There is no evidence that these patterns represent any drastic change from the near past.

Another discrepancy in the centenarian lineages was revealed by Arlene Hoffman, the chief researcher for the Dannon yogurt commercials made in the U.S.S.R.[10] Her colleagues in New York City had conceived of a commercial showing a centenarian eating yogurt with the approval of his or her mother or father. Because the traditional link between yogurt and longevity had been associated with Bulgaria, the first attempt to find such a parent–sibling pairing was made through that country's government. After unsuccessful internal inquiries, the Bulgarians suggested that Hoffman might do better in the Soviet Union. The assistance of officials in Moscow, Kiev, Tbilisi, and Sukhumi was obtained, but the best combination that could be found was Bagrat Topagua, age 89, and his mother, Warde, age 117. Apparently not one of the 500 supercentenarians could produce a nonagenarian, much less a centenarian, offspring.

Some Azerbaijan doctors have advanced the theory that longevity may be related to small family units occurring within patterns of a slowed life cycle marked by delayed menarche and delayed menopause in women. Sula Benet has reproduced a list of 8 multigenerational Azerbaijan families offered as possible proof of this idea.[11] Though this is described as a list of people having "many offspring," there is only 1 five-generational example. It stems from a woman reputed to be 120 and having 236 descendants. The other 7 cases cite individuals aged 101 to 130 having offspring through four generations numbering from 38 to 53! The 2 men included are said to have fathered children at 93 and 104 respectively, and some of the women are said to have given birth after age 60.

These claims are at odds with official Soviet health records. As Gogoghian pointed out, births after the mid-40s are rare, and none has been accepted for a woman older than 55. As for family size, the 1959 census established the average Azerbaijan family as 4.5 persons, with 161 families out of every thousand having 7 or more members. The figures are similar in Georgia (4.0 and 84) and Armenia (4.8 and 194). These are much *higher*, not lower, than findings for the Baltic republics, the Soviet areas with the lowest longevity. There, the average family size ranged from a low of 3.1 in Estonia, with 14 households per thousand having 7 or more members, to a high of 3.6 in Lithuania, with 43 households per thousand having 7 or more members.[12] The thesis is further undercut by the Kiev observation that women in the age group 80–104 had borne *twice as many* children as had women in the age group 60–79.[13] Like so much of the Azerbaijan-derived data, the linkage of longevity to late marriages, small families, and delayed biological cycles is a circular argument necessitated by the very oral histories it hopes to substantiate and demanding exceptionalism from centenarian data available elsewhere in the U.S.S.R. and abroad.

A far more plausible theory accounting for the limited number of offspring and generations is that many of the long-living have falsified their ages by from ten to thirty years. Putting in this correction would dissolve the generation gap for all but the most extravagant age claims and would mean that just as elsewhere in the world, great- and great-great grandparents would be in their late 80s, 90s, and early 100s. The total number of offspring would also make more statistical sense.

Another difficulty with the supercentenarian data that

Soviet gerontologists have not addressed adequately is the mathematical irregularities posed. If, for instance, Shirali Mislimov was actually 168 at his death, and Makhum Ayvazov, the previously recognized oldest person, was 156 at the time of his death, there is a gerontological chasm of a dozen years between them.[14] This compares with the mere ninety days separating Pierre Joubert from Delina Filkins. As soon as anyone over 120 is accepted as verified, comparable gaps appear for age categories going back to at least the late 90s, where Medvedev has already identified significant irregularities of a different nature. Given the falling rate of centenarianism between 1959 and 1970 and the projected decline in the forthcoming census, the possibility of discovering more longevous people, particularly centenarians and supercentenarians, is quite bleak.

Further evidence that falsification, particularly of the higher claims, is at the root of the statistical dilemma can be discerned in Georgian specifics. Of the 1,844 centenarians of 1970, there were 1,230 women and 614 men. Proceeding at five-year intervals, the 2–1 ratio of women to men remains constant through age 115. From that point through age 119, there is a 3–2 ratio of 34 women to 20 men. In the ages above 120, however, there is cataclysmic reversal, with 42 surviving men and only 20 women.[15] This statistical improbability is best explained as a result of the patriarchs' bragging about their ages and their exaggerations being recorded as fact. Official unease with these figures is indicated by the lumping of all supercentenarians into one category rather than continuation of the five-year-interval method used to chart the other 1,782 centenarians.

Still more devastating signs of sexist fraud are found when the longest-living women are compared with the longest-living men. Allowing Khfaf Lazuria the luxury of 140 years, there remain hundreds of men claiming to have outlived her and an incredible twenty-eight years separating her from Mislimov. Since everywhere in the world centenarian women outnumber centenarian men by at least 2 to 1 and since there is commingling of the sexes in that ratio in every age group through 115, even in Georgia, the sudden sex gap is intolerable.

The flimsy nature of the supercentenarian claims reflects poorly on the oral-history verifications, which, owing to the lack of primary sources, must remain the heart of Soviet field work. The staggering diversity of languages and cultures in the Soviet Union, the massive illiteracy of most of those born before the Revolution, and the difficulty of year-round access to mountain regons have already been cited as formidable verification obstacles. Professionals doing oral histories in simpler contexts know that a considerable amount of time is required to do the job correctly. One cannot just walk in and take notes or run a tape recorder for half an hour and then go on to another centenarian. Second and third visits are essential to clear up ambiguities and other problems that will not be evident until the original material has been studied. The whole account, in turn, needs to be judged for accuracy against all other available materials. The centenarians to be interviewed numbered roughly 20,000 persons. If only eight hours were spent on each person, a quarter-million hours, or six thousand forty-hour weeks, would be needed to complete the task. Finding field workers with the proper historical knowledge, language skills, and interviewing techniques to do such investigations would be a major undertaking in itself, even if computers were available to facilitate the tabulation of data. As it is, local physicians not necessarily trained in social sciences have done most of the verifications personally or through subordinates representing a wide range of backgrounds.

Virtually all the proofs found in the oral histories made available to Westerners can be reduced to a matter of trust in the word of the particular respondent. When a venerable points to a mark on the wall of his home and insists his father made it one hundred and thirty years ago to record his birth, one can believe or disbelieve. How many interviewers will have the intellectual courage to challenge such an assertion, especially in cultures where respect for elders is so intense? Likewise an inscription in a Koran or a Bible may indicate the birth of one Makhtil Targil, but living in the same compound are Makhtil Targil I, II, and III. There were preceding Makhtil Targils in earlier generations and cousins of the same or similar name. Recalling that there was no alphabet for Abkhasian before the Revolution and illiteracy ran to 98 percent, the room for error is considerable. The rarely available church record may be authentic, but to whom does it refer? Assessing the truth in oral histories is further complicated by the rigid customs regulating male–female exchanges and by ethnic pride.

A major assumption in the oral-history approach is that the questions are so chronologically mixed that a falsifier could not sustain consistency. But this mistakes illiteracy for lack of mental acumen. Peasants have always done complicated sums in their heads, and they can juggle dates as nimbly as can university graduates. Nor must it be assumed they do not know the Great Snow fell in 1910 or that the emancipation of the serfs in Abkhasia took place in 1870 (nine years later than in Russia proper, another opportunity for error to occur). Khfaf Lazuria's accounts were all internally consistent and were supported by family and neighbors. Discrepancies appeared only through a comparison of stories told at different times.

Vagueness is another shortcoming. Kamachich Kavichenya claimed to have been kidnapped during the Turkish raids. This could be any time between 1858 and 1878, with the question of exactly how young she was a matter to be settled solely at her discretion. When pressed to explain how the incident demonstrated she was 137 and not 117, she explained that she was in pigtails when taken in one of the first raids. Assuming she was not lying, what does "first" mean? First for her village? For her region? For the whole era? How could she even know? Ten to twenty years could accrue to someone's age by a misdating of such episodes. Often too, the personal details of life are related to famous historical events. But it is just these events which are most vividly recounted in the area's strong oral traditions. Many of the oldest of the long-living are consistently referred to as raconteurs, musicians, and storytellers. Their ability to fashion credible fictitious histories should be self-evident. There also can be no doubt that at least some of the long-living are no longer sure whether they heard about the great war in the North at the time it happened or whether it was a story handed down by parents and grandparents. Locating the historical truth in this maze of confusion, legend, deceit, and vanity depends in great measure on the attitudes of the investigators. Are they, like Sula Benet, eager to believe? Or are they a doubting Thoms?

Soviet researchers have been candid in acknowledging the inherent difficulties of the oral-history verifications, and they make revisions constantly. After the original 1959 census identified 29,000 centenarians, 8,000 were totally eliminated by follow-up investigations, for a correction of over 25 percent. Checks of the 1970 census results in Georgia dealt with 2,681 longevity claims and showed that 836 individuals had inflated their ages by from three to ten years and another 77 had inflated them by more than ten years, for a total downward correction of 35 percent. There were also 120 persons (a little over 4 percent who had understated their ages.[16] Investigations of specific cases indicate that the incidence and magnitude of error increased as the age advanced beyond 109 into superlongevous territory. If highly trained persons redid the interviews, it is certain the number of centenarians per 100,000 of population would be substantially reduced. But even with such reductions, the overall longevity rate in the Caucasus would most likely remain the highest in the world.

The supercentenarian claims are another matter. In view of the percentage of distortion, the vagueness of the oral histories, and the statistical abnormalities, none of them can be accepted as proved. If Soviet officials still believe the claims are valid, there is a relatively simple way to resolve international doubts. Detailed oral histories, physical-test results, genealogical charts, generational photographs, autopsy reports (when available), and other proofs of the 10 or 20 best cases could be presented to an international blue-ribbon committee convened in a spirit of cooperative inquiry rather than nationalist or ideological conflict. These experts could be given the freedom to verify or reject the claims by all recognized methods. Since they would be the best claims available, with the preliminary work done by Soviet experts, the verification process could be relatively swift. Regardless of the outcome, the launching of such a project would be a kind of gerontological Sputnik for which the Soviet Union could only be lauded. If, as is likely, the claims were judged invalid, Soviet gerontologists would be relieved of the super-centenarian burden, which casts such a negative shadow over their otherwise considerable achievement. On the other hand, should even one supercentenarian be verified, it would be as significant to biology as the splitting of the atom was to physics and would call for a fundamental rethinking of present givens. The chances for such an inquiry are slim, for there is every indication that supercentenarians are no longer taken seriously by the leading Soviet experts. The strongest signal is that the major emphasis in antiaging research has shifted from the study of centenarians to projects that rely heavily on medical intervention.

The most monumental of the new longevity programs is Project 2000, begun by Chebotarev and his associates in 1970.[17] It involves 2,000 urban dwellers who range in age from the early 20s to the 90s. All have agreed to follow regimens set up for them by the gerontologists and to take periodic physical examinations, which are more frequent for the oldest participants. The specifics of the program are secret, but its components are psychological counseling, diet control, exercise programs, and chemical intervention. The last involves vitamins, hormones, and antioxidants. The volunteers are divided so that each combination of therapies is used by a portion of each age group. The de facto control group for Project 2000 is the general Soviet public as measured by the average life-span, but among the volunteers there are those whose pills and injections are placebos. Any longevity gain on their part would have to be attributed to psychosomatic factors or the regular medical checkups.

The part of the project most directly linked to the field studies is the counseling area. There are lectures and discussions to teach families how to interact more positively with their older members, while the older people are given guidance on how to remain reasonably self-sufficient for as long as possible. Additional work, done with everyone, seeks to show why the particular exercises suggested are thought to be prolongevous. The researchers have discovered that, just like the Abkhasians, many of the volunteers state that they now expect to live to be at least one hundred. Quite a few add that just being part of the project has given them a long-term psychological uplift, for they feel their lives have taken on historical importance.

Taking a different experimental direction from Chebotarev's are scientists organized in the late 1970s into the National Committee for the Artificial Prolongation of Human Life.[18] The vice-chairman of the group and a biologist at the Institute of General Genetics is Dr. L. V. Komarov. He believes that within the next hundred years, methods will be found to extend life to from three to four hundred years, and that life extension may go to one hundred fifty years in the near future. He speaks of slowing down the aging process through drug combinations. His own work has centered on adenosine triphosphate (ATP), an enzyme found in greater quantities in the bodies of the young than in the old. ATP is currently used in the Soviet Union to help ward off disease, and Komarov believes that in combination with other substances, it may be a key antiaging weapon. Studies already in hand have determined that used alone, ATP cannot retard aging. Komarov, who at 59 looks to be in his early 40s, is rumored to have used himself as an experimental subject, but officially, his work prior to 1978 was confined to insects.

Using magnetized sugar and other macroenergetic substances, he has doubled the life-span of houseflies. Set up in a
new laboratory with five assistants, in the 1980s Komarov
will work with human volunteers. Other research on the
artificial prolongation of life done elsewhere in the U.S.S.R.
will be coordinated through the National Committee. In
Odessa, for example, the Filatov Institute has been con-
ducting experiments using an extract from human placentas
preserved after childbirth.

Experiments of this kind are not without precedents,
albeit unsuccessful ones, in the Soviet Union. At the out-
break of World War II, Dr. Alexander A. Bogomoletz, the
founder of the Kiev Institute and a pioneer in the investigation of centenarian claims, announced that he had developed
a vaccine (antireticular cytotoxic serum) which seemed to
prolong life. The work was interrupted by the war, and when
it resumed in the late 1940s, the claim was withdrawn. In the
mid-'50s a new combination called Gerovital which had been
devised by Dr. Ana Aslan of Rumania was thought capable of
revitalizing the body, but although Dr. Aslan reported that
older people brought to her clinic for treatment were rejuvenated, tests undertaken in several other nations failed to
reproduce her results. Among those who have been widely
rumored to have used the drug without apparent success were
Nikita Khrushchev, Konrad Adenauer, and Mao Tse-tung.

The basis of Aslan's formula is procaine hydrochloride—
or as it is more commonly known in the United States,
novocaine. She has added benzoic acid, a preservative, and
potassium metabisulfate, an antioxidant. Her injections are
given in conjunction with megavitamin treatments and close
monitoring of the patients' vital signs. Zhores Medvedev
thinks the disparities between her results and those obtained
by others is due to the source of her patients.[19] Rumania has
one of Europe's lowest average life-spans and one of its lowest
standards of living. Aslan's patients are mainly sickly pensioners taken from old-age homes where treatment is not up
to the standards of developed nations. The attention given to

the pensioners, the vitamins, the good food, the proper exercise, and the comfortable surroundings, Medvedev argues, account for their improved health. He professes that testing in Kiev proved that Gerovital is worthless and that that led to the U.S.S.R.'s abandoning it. Aslan has claimed that incorrect combinations were used in the tests done outside Rumania, but it is inconceivable that the Soviets would not have been able to obtain and would not have used her exact procedures and formulas. In spite of the failure to reproduce her results anywhere else, a health cult has emerged around Aslan's work. In major American cities, Gerovital is sold clandestinely as a "forbidden" youth drug, and Rumanian advertisements seeking to attract American tourists shamelessly suggest that three points of interest are the Carpathian Mountains, Dracula's castle, and "the youth clinics of Dr. Ana Aslan."[20]

Quite distinct from the chemotherapy approach and borrowing from longevity field studies is the Soviet infatuation with the sanitariums and health spas available for vacations. Rest, diet control, mineral baths, weight loss, and pleasant surroundings are part of a proletarianized version of what the nineteenth-century bourgeoisie referred to as "the cure." The major area for activity of this kind is the coast of the Black Sea, including, of late, Abkhasia. Other vacation spots include the coast of the Caspian Sea, where, in Baku, a program called the Zone of Health, operated by the Health Spa System under the Ministry of Health, has caught the fancy of American observers looking for longevity regimens based on natural therapies.[21]

The Zone of Health concept is the brainchild of Dr. Shukyur Gasanov, who launched the program in the summer of 1961. By the 1970s over 150,000 people were coming to the Baku center annually, and new facilities were being constructed to accommodate the 250,000 annual visitors anticipated in the 1980s. The program involves a six-week effort aimed at adding eight to ten years to a person's life—"full, satisfying years," as Gasanov likes to say. Strictly forbidden in the Zone of Health is the use of medication of any sort. Instead, the backbone of the program is group exercise such as rhythmic walking, rhythmic breathing, calisthenics at the beach, dancing, and swimming, all augmented by massages and water therapy. The beach activities begin early in the morning and continue at various times throughout the day even if it is drizzling.

The Zone, which is free to retirees and available at nominal cost to workers, attracts an older population. Gasanov likes to have them chant, "We are not a burden" as part of their psychological orientation. Other activities of the same nature include group singing. Melancholy songs are discouraged by the effervescent Gasanov, who insists on tunes that are "boisterous and vigorous." Far more unusual and possibly verging on quackery is Gasanov's unique contribution to longevity therapy, fiotherapy: the systematic sniffing of flowers and herbs thought to be prolongevous. This was inspired by his study of Azerbaijan folk remedies and includes rosemary, flowering laurel, Baku sandalwood, and geraniums. In the future, Gasanov plans to have separate sniffing chambers which will be bathed in hues designed to soothe the patient's emotions.

Henry Gris has called Gasanov the Guru of Baku and the Zone of Health a California on the Caspian. Certainly the overweight and bucolic Gasanov seems more like the social director of a jolly holiday camp than a health maven. Yet his basic ideas make sense. The emphasis on exercise and a fat-free diet could not be better. The immediate benefits of the program to overweight, depressed, or sedentary people can be considerable. Most of the other activities, fiotherapy, singing, and chanting included, fuse into one enormous ego-building effort constructed on the assumption that a pleasant disposition and an appetite for life are critical for any prolongevous agenda. While not in the same heavyweight division as the work in Kiev done by Chebotarev and his associates or that coordinated by Komarov, the Zone of Health is a decent and credible attempt to put some gerontological knowledge to immediate use. The main drawback, as Gasanov will admit, is that the changes might be temporary. Six weeks of healthful living cannot make up for forty-six of abuse, and the longevity prospects of an octogenarian depend in large measure on how he or she has chosen to live during most of the preceding decades, not on a few weeks snatched for health here and there. One might also question how effective the Zone would be without the infectious enthusiasm of its originator.

What is striking about the age goals set for the various longevity projects is that they aim only for approximately 100 years of life. Komarov states unequivocally that without the development of appropriate chemical combinations or medical procedures, the limit of life will remain less than 120.[22] This attitude is reflected in persons as diverse as Chebotarev, Gasanov, and Gogoghian. With this in mind, the superlongevous range of 110–114 established as the outer limit of achieved life for documented centenarians is not materially altered by Soviet findings.

The thrust of the new longevity work further indicates that the Soviets have concluded that the direct study of centenarians has already exhausted most of what can be learned through that method alone. While ongoing centenarian work continues to be a concern, rather than yielding new fundamentals, such efforts are likely to refine factors already found in the encyclopedic work of the 1960s and '70s. To get large numbers of people into the centenarian ranks and to strike out for new age highs, the Soviets have turned to artificial means for prolonging life. The risky nature of this work can be appreciated by the fact that estrogen injections, which once were thought to have a rejuvenating effect on women, have been shown to encourage cancers and heart disease. Similar negative side effects may result from substances being investigated by the Soviet researchers. It is always an awesome decision to move from apparently successful work with laboratory cultures and other forms of life to work with human volunteers. The Soviets are taking that bold step in the effort to extend and enhance life. If they succeed, the supercentenarian barrier may at last fall. Until then, to find a human being who has seen a thirteenth decade, we must look elsewhere.

4

LONGEVITY IN THE MOUNTAINS

> Vilcabamba is in a hollow in the
> mountains where five valleys con-
> verge and, seen from above, looks
> like the arms of a star, Vilcabamba
> being in the center . . .
>
> —*David Davies*

Mountain regions have always bred legends of long-living
people. The explanation most commonly advanced in national literatures is that the harsh weather conditions and the
physical exertion required for simple survival have produced
men and women surefooted, ornery, and sturdy as the hoofed
and horned animals with which they share the heights. As
postwar interest in the Soviet Caucasus grew, gerontologists
turned to these stories to see if areas with similar topography
might not also contain longevous populations. In widely
scattered regions of the world, the connection between
mountain terrain and long life was promising. The most
exciting prospects involved the Vilcabamba Valley of south-
eastern Ecuador, where supercentenarian claims were backed
by religious and civil records.

Vilcabamba enjoys a historical association with good
health dating back to Inca times, but its most recent fame

began in the 1950s when heart specialists wrote about the impressive cardiovascular vigor of its inhabitants. Popular interest was fanned by a spirited 1956 press conference in New York City featuring Javier Pereira, a man reputed to be 167, who had been brought to the United States by the owners of a syndicated newspaper feature titled *Believe It or Not.*[1] Fifteen years later came the sensational news that a census had found 9 centenarians in a village of 819 persons. If accurate, this number would give Vilcabamba a centenarian population nearly 400 times that of the United States and nearly 30 times that of Soviet Georgia. This was all the more remarkable as Vilcabamba was in one of the poorest areas of South America, where health facilities were inadequate, hygiene poorly understood, and social relations strained by a brutal feudalistic economy.

Dr. David Davies of the Gerontological Unit, University College, London, was among the most enthusiastic boosters of the Vilcabamba claims. Aided by a number of Ecuadorian scientists and with some technical help from various levels of the Ecuadorian government, Davies made four visits to the valley between 1971 and 1973. The main evidence for longevity he found was a series of records kept by the Roman Catholic churches.[2] They stretched back to the eighteenth century, and their authenticity was beyond dispute. The records were far more substantial than any documentation available in the Caucasus, and there were civil records going back to 1900 which could be used as a cross-reference.

Davies questioned many of the reputed superlongevous. A person who particularly impressed him was the oldest of the Vilcabamba centenarians, Miguel Carpio, who claimed to be 123. Satisfied with the documentation presented, Davies thought Carpio to be "very lucid" and took down a description of the Peruvian War of 1894 in which Carpio claimed to have fought. Three old women in the village, one of them a centenarian herself, remembered Carpio as already grown when they were still children. A number of men who attested to Carpio's age also claimed to be in the superlongevous category.[3] The cluster of interrelated verifications and re-membered historical events was similar to those encountered in the Caucasus.

Observations of life in Vilcabamba and the immediate area were to turn up a number of discordant elements, which Davies recorded but did not consider critical. For example, many of the men smoked from one to forty cigarettes a day, and on Saturday nights it was common for men to drink steadily until they passed out. Nonetheless, there were numerous male centenarians, and after age 105 they far outnumbered the women. Another element not found in other observations of long-living people was the social dis-tance between generations. Speaking of specific centenarian families, Davies wrote, "They did not seem particularly close to their children or vice versa. They would meet each other regularly after church on Sunday morning but other meetings were not frequent."[4]

Rather than pursue these matters, Davies concentrated his study on the physical environment. He determined that the critical feature of Vilcabamba was that the soil was unusually rich in minerals, particularly selenium. This fitted his already formed hypothesis that trace elements might be critical to longevity. However, the accuracy of his tests cannot be accepted at face value, because his writing demon-strated a marked penchant for exaggeration and inaccuracy. He suggested, for instance, that "Any heart patient, from any part of the world, improves after a visit to the village."[5] Trying to compare Vilcabamba to Abkhasia, he reported erroneously that there were 150,000 Abkhasians instead of the 500,000 of the 1970 census and 2,000 reputed cente-narians instead of the actual 294. He thought Shirali Mis-limov was an Abkhasian and seemed oblivious to the distinctions between Georgia, Azerbaijan, and Abkhasia.[6] All in all, his work was more like that of a mythologizer than that of a scientist and was important mainly for the attention it directed to the church and civil documentation.

Equally excited about Vilcabamba was Grace Halsell, an

author who lived in Ecuador for most of 1974 and spent considerable time in Vilcabamba. Halsell has made a career of changing identities in order to write books about specific cultures. She dyed her skin black and lived as a black woman in Harlem and Mississippi for one book and lived as an illegal Mexican alien for another project. She could not age for Vilcabamba, but she thought the length of time she spent living in the area as an ordinary inhabitant would give her work a poignancy and authenticity brief visits lacked. Her experiences were recorded in *Los Viejos*, published in 1976 by Rodale press, a major publisher of health books in the United States.

Like Davies, Halsell made a point of searching out the records and described herself as "a little awed" by the age of the documents.[7] Her only other attempts at verification were the usual ones in which individuals in at least their 70s remembered that the centenarians had already been "old" when they were "young." Her explanation for Vilcabamba longevity did not stray far beyond the organic-food, pollution-free, natural-life-style approach advocated in the pages of *Prevention* and *Organic Gardening*, the best-known publications issued by her book publisher.

Halsell also made a stab at social analysis that is typical of the illusions often spread about underdeveloped areas with reputedly longevous inhabitants. Not finding the kind of tension and stress common in developed nations, she believed that the people Frantz Fanon characterized as the wretched of the earth—the social base that has fed one contemporary revolutionary movement after another—achieved longevity because of the serene nature of their life-style. Like a nineteenth-century liberal commentator on American slavery, she wrote, "I could see the evils of the hacienda system and would, under no circumstances, exchange my life for the role of a peon. Yet, I also noted the *viejos* had used their harsh circumstances to build strong, good characters . . . It seemed ironic that the *viejos*, among the poorest people of the world, would worry less about money and possessions than the richest people in the world."[8] Brushing aside her own anecdotes of sexual passion, jealousies, violence, and anger, Halsell canonized the old with observations that "A *viejo* does not hate, he is not bitter"[9] and "I have never heard them quarrel or fight or dispute with each other."[10]

Such romanticization does not stand up when compared with detailed Vilcabamba biographies of longevous people, who invariably display all the normal human reactions to pain and adversity. The notion that poverty somehow produces strong character, physical fitness, and mental health is a delusion. The massive outmigration of young people from underdeveloped mountain areas is a clear demonstration of how they feel, and that the effects of poverty on the old can be as devastating in the Andean hut as they are in the North American rooming house has been amply documented.[11]

The somber realities of Andean poverty made a deep impression on Alexander Leaf, who visited Vilcabamba in 1970 and again in 1974. Even though he accepted the authenticity of the church records, his studies of the centenarians left him puzzled. The terrain, the low cholesterol level in the blood, and the meager daily 1,200-calorie intake might explain the low incidence of heart disease, but such factors were found throughout the mountains. There were also the numerous negative factors already cited. Leaf came to lean toward the thesis that whatever longevity existed was a product of genetics. The Vilcabambans were of a slightly different ethnic line than most of the neighboring people, and many of the longevous were blood relatives.[12]

Leaf was aware, too, of specific exaggerations of age. A brother of Miguel Carpio who claimed to be 122 on the 1970 visit had zoomed to 134 four years later.[13] José David Toledo, who told Leaf that he was 107 in 1970, claimed to *The New York Times* to be 141 in 1973.[14] Leaf thought a detailed examination of the church and civil records might be profitable.

The challenge was taken up by Dr. Sylvia H. Forman, a

specialist in quantitative anthropology, and Dr. Richard B. Mazess, who wanted to determine the rate of calcium loss in the bones of the longevous. In 1974 they conducted a survey of the skeletal status of the longevous and did a household census which involved 80 percent of the population. The church records and civil registry were examined after family genealogies had been worked out. In 1976 and 1978, Mazess returned for further work. A familiar longevity hoax emerged: the records of older relatives had been appropriated by younger people, sons taking the records of fathers and nieces taking the records of aunts.[15] Some false claims were the result of honest confusion and semiliteracy, but many, particularly the supercentenarian claims of the men, were conscious deceptions. Of the 9 centenarians of the 1971 census, none was genuine. The oldest in the group was 96, and some were only septuagenarians.

Miguel Carpio's falsifications were typical. Because of the similarity of family names, various records had become confused, and the local officials came to believe he was born in 1864, which led to the official age of 112 recorded at the time of his death in 1976. This already cut some fifteen years off his top age claim, but methodical work by Mazess and Forman was to take off another nineteen. It was established that Carpio's mother had been born in 1855 and that he had been born in 1883. Seven other entries between 1905 and 1915 made the identifications conclusive. For Carpio to have been 127 in 1976, he would have needed to be born six years before his mother, and for him to be 112, would have meant that his mother had given birth at age 9. Still more entries established that he began to lie about his age in 1944, when he claimed to be 70 while only 61. Five years later his age had jumped to 80.

With the linchpin of Carpio pulled, all the claims interconnected with his tumbled as well. However, Mazess and Forman went beyond such circumstantial evidence. They were able to locate records for nearly all of the longevous claimants. Their conclusions stunned the gerontologists and faddists who had wanted to accept Vilcabamban stories: "None of the 23 'centenarians' investigated had, in fact, survived to 100 years. Similarly, none of the 15 'non-agenarians' investigated had, in fact, survived 90 years."[16] The very records that had once been the bulwark of the claims now disproved them. An important element in the deverifications was the genealogies worked out by Forman which made it possible to sort out the family relationships.

A significant ancillary discovery was that exaggerations of age had been a tradition since at least the turn of the century, so that the postwar tourist and scientific interest only fed an established custom. The apparently high concentration of older people was another illusion. Its cause was the mass exodus of young people to the cities, leaving depopulated villages with deceptively high numbers of abandoned old people. Without a massive demographic study, no absolute judgments could be made, but Mazess and Forman were confident about the conclusions to be drawn from their efforts: "Individual longevity in Vilcabamba is little, if any, different from that found throughout the rest of the world."[17]

Fortunately, as is so often the case in longevity hoaxes involving studies of large populations, the research in Vilcabamba had not been entirely fruitless in establishing useful data about the nature of aging. At a conference held in 1978, Japanese, French, Canadian, Ecuadorian, and American scientists correlated the Vilcabamba research they had done independently. The conferees agreed that the over-70 population in Vilcabamba had unusual cardiovascular health. Some indications of this were their low blood pressure, their low heart rates after exertion, and the finding that they had only one-third of the cardiac abnormalities usually found in the same age categories in developed nations. Their cardiovascular health appeared to be linked to their leanness, their diet, their low cholesterol levels, and their high level of physical activity. It was found also that the older Vilcabambans were relatively free of the symptoms of aging (spinal curvature, pain, fractures) associated with osteoporosis.[18]

The scope of the Vilcabamba hoax is sobering for anyone wishing to give the benefit of the doubt to undocumented claims supported only by oral histories and local traditions. In this case, the longevity myth was rooted in the low rate of cancer and heart diseases in the area. Upon this factual base, some Ecuadorian officials had hoped that Vilcabamba might be transformed into a health resort. Writers, publishers, and scientists eager to find their pet theories proved added their own distortions. In response to this attention, the inhabitants made the most of their possibilities, gaining relief from the tedium of their existence and perhaps hopeful of some financial reward or a trip to the United States. As elsewhere, men were more brazen in their lies than women, and there was a tendency for baffled observers to believe the population might possess unique genetic inheritance.

Another area in the Western Hemisphere frequently thought to be prolongevous is the hot and arid Sierra Madre range of northern Mexico. The region's most celebrated inhabitants are the Tarahumara Indians, a people who have the distinction of being the world's only jogging nation. Their name can be roughly translated as "foot runners," and foot running is their basic means of travel and the basis of their sports. *Run, don't walk* would be an apt national motto for them.

Tarahumara hunters can chase deer for two and three days on end until the animal either drops from exhaustion or is run over the edge of a ravine. The stalking involves considerable tracking and walking, but long stretches of jogging are an essential ingredient of the kill. Even more common among the Tarahumara are footraces, the national pastime. In 1928 two Tarahumara men, José Torres and Aurelio Terrazas, took part in the Olympic marathon competition held in Amsterdam. They lost first place by several minutes, but claimed they had thought the race was going to be much longer or they would have run faster. Another Tarahumara sport is a kickball game which is played over a range of from two to a dozen miles and can last from noon to sunset. Occasionally some games are said to go on for a period of days.

Physical endurance of this nature would be impressive in any terrain, but it is doubly so in the Sierra Madre, one of the least hospitable environments in North America. Its demanding climate and poor soil make the continuing existence of Tarahumara culture a kind of ecological marvel. Even though the major crops of corn, pumpkins, and beans were often in short supply and most Tarahumara still did not speak Spanish, in the 1970s the group numbered 40,000.

Owing to the enthusiasm for jogging in the adjacent United States, legends about Tarahumara longevity have multiplied. The verification problem, however, is even more difficult than in Azerbaijan. In the 1930s, long before the American jogging craze, Wendell Bennett and Robert Zingle made an anthropological survey of Tarahumara culture. They discovered that while the tribal language had words for "day" and "week," the word for "month" was the same as that for "moon," and the year was only crudely reckoned by the position of the sun in the sky in relation to certain fixed points. The Tarahumara did not know how many days were in a month or how many months were in a year. They did not have names for individual months, and they did not bother to keep track of years.[19] Thus, any statement that a Tarahumara has lived a hundred years must be speculative.

Noticeable by its absence in the Bennet-and-Zingle work is any reference to large numbers of old people or the hint of longevity. What was striking to the anthropologists was the low level of medical knowledge and basic hygiene. They were told many plants could cure bruises and abrasions, but the injuries they saw were usually neglected, and the most minor skin breaks could lead to severe infections.

Some forty years after the investigation of Bennet and Zingle, a *National Geographic* team reported on another antilongevous aspect of the culture: the musical and drinking feasts known as the *tutuguri*. One of these affairs was described as ". . . a cacophony of chanting, fiddles, rattles, guitars, stomping dances, shouts, raucous laughter, and howling dogs. Both men and women dropped out to drink corn beer (they rarely drink anything stronger) and soon were staggering about in a stupor."[20] The commentator, James Norman, goes on to call the massive drunkenness a "strange and sad phenomenon."[21] He judged that each Tarahumara spent about one hundred days a year preparing, drinking, and recovering from corn beer, with some individuals taking part in as many as ninety parties. A minimum of two hundred pounds of corn per family was estimated to be needed for the preparation of corn beer annually, even though the usage cut into the already minimal food supply. This alcoholic abuse would likely neutralize all the health gains accrued through jogging even without the other negative factors of poor healing skills and a diet hovering around malnutrition.

Even more disappointing than the Vilcabamba and Sierra Madre studies have been investigations dealing with the Carpathian Mountains. In the Soviet sector of the range no significant longevity was found,[22] and in the Rumanian sector the rates were lower than those found among West European city dwellers.[23] The Rumanian study, done in the 1960s, is still important, however, because it identified longevity factors similar to those in the Caucasus. Patterning its work on the Soviet models, the Rumanian government sponsored a study of 5,123 persons over 85 years of age. Instead of mountaineers, agricultural workers made up 54 percent of the group, the lumpy category of housewives another 24 percent, and then manual workers. Most of these individuals had done the same kind of work for most of their lives, and few had ever formally retired. Thirty-five percent were lactovegetarians and 5 percent were primarily fish eaters, with the rest consuming a mixed diet. Thirty-eight percent reported that neither parent was longevous, and 16 percent did not know. One unusual finding was that in the group over 95, 20 percent were primarily fish eaters. This group also had the lowest number of bedridden persons. The researchers did not determine how much this phenomenon was due to diet and how much was related to the arduous life of the sea. The study further determined that 77 percent of those over 85 and 95 percent of those over 95 had never smoked.

Yet another study which produced results similar to the longevity profile found in the Caucasus was done in the 1970s.[24] This time the target was a mountain region of Turkey, and the investigators, Suha Beller and Erdman Palmore, were less concerned with the percentages of lon-gevous people and verifying ages than with making detailed biographical sketches. They located 50 individuals claiming to be over 90 and 13 claiming to be over 100. Although documentation was lacking, the investigators were confident that all the participants were at least octogenarians. Again, the cluster of longevity factors resembled those in the U.S.S.R. The long-living ate very simple diets with little meat or animal fat. They had body types described as being from normal to lean, but definitely much leaner than that of the general population. The long-living also had a vigorous life-style, exemplified by one man who insisted on walking at least 5 miles a day as a health measure. Eighty-six percent of the group had never smoked, and only 4 percent had ever smoked more than a pack of cigarettes a day.

Social relationships were similar to those in the Cau-casus as well. All had been married at least once, and they related to extended family networks in which they held honored and secure positions. While the social prestige was not as formalized as in the Caucasus, it was considerable. Most likely as a result of this psychological support, the group was found to have a positive mental outlook and a high rate of social ability.

A number of biochemical tests constituted another aspect of the survey. Eighty-six percent of those seen were judged to be in good health, with only 14 percent house-bound. Vision and hearing were generally good. The only unusual results were some common blood factors. Since the sampling was so small, the investigators did not think it wise to form any generalization, and subsequent work dealing with blood factors remains inconclusive.

Tracking down the tales of longevity in the mountains sometimes appears to be little more than an exercise in debunking, but this isn't so. The studies of mountain people have revealed that significant benefits to the cardiovascular, respiratory, and skeletal systems can be derived from rugged terrain. The advantages to the heart and lungs are linked to the thinness of the air at higher altitudes and the constant physical challenge of walking on inclines. The process is comparable to the way a biceps is built up through the repeated strain of lifting an iron bar. The cardiovascular and respiratory health of mountain people of every age also indicates that heart diseases are not an inexorable fate for those in the 50–90 age bracket. As the majority of people in the developed world suffer from heart diseases while in that age spectrum, it is possible to hypothesize that sedentary populations presently suffer from an epidemic of premature and preventable deaths not unlike the premature deaths once caused by infectious diseases.

Such a view finds support in numerous studies of occupations and activity patterns. Among the best-known is a survey involving 31,000 London transport workers. Heart diseases were much more frequent among the drivers of double-decker buses than among ticket takers on the same buses, who walked back and forth and up and down the bus stairs all day.[25] A Finnish study discovered that woodcutters live seven to eight years longer than office workers.[26] An American study that compared a group of male Irish immigrants in Boston with their brothers still in Ireland found the Irish siblings to be longer-living. The primary difference was that in Ireland the men had to walk or cycle several miles a day to agricultural jobs, while in the United States the men used motorized transportation to reach city jobs of various descriptions.[27] Other studies of 17,000 college graduates,[28] 6,551 stevedores,[29] 16,882 office workers,[30] and 119,000 postal carriers[31] have shown similar positive correlations between longer life and strenuous physical activity.

Exercise also confers great benefits on the skeletal system. In the mountains, a tougher system less subject to fracture seems to be due to the stimulation of the bone marrow caused by walking and climbing. Just moving about mountainous terrain accomplishing daily survival tasks is equivalent to hours of formal exercise. Like heart disease, fragile bones, the curse of so many aging Americans, result more from lack of conditioning than from the mere passage of time.

The mountain studies thus provide useful evidence that calendar age is less significant than biological or physiological age, which in turn is highly dependent upon the kinds of physical demands made on the body. At the same time, the studies demonstrate that terrain, altitude, and exercise in and of themselves are not a sufficient combination to produce unusual longevity. To them must be added the dietary and psychological factors found in the Caucasus, and there must be no horrendously negative habits like alcoholism or cigarette smoking.

Authentic centenarians may yet be found in the Sierra Madre, the Andes, and the Carpathians. Certainly there is evidence that healthy octogenarian and nonagenarian individuals may be found in higher percentages there than in less demanding geographic zones. It is predictable that the belief in the wholesale longevity of mountain people and the existence of supercentenarians among them will persist until the respective governments become interested enough in vital statistics to devise systems for gathering accurate data. Someone will suggest that if Vilcabamba doesn't have centenarians, then other Andean villages do. Or if the Tarahumara visited by the *National Geographic* are drunkards, the more traditional groups deeper in the mountains are not. The supercentenarian haven will always be in that neglected valley over the horizon.

5

THE HUNZAKUTS

> The point of Gilgit, now as always, is strategic. High above the snow-line, somewhere midst the peaks and glaciers that wall in the Gilgit valley, the long and jealously guarded frontiers of India, China, Russia, Afghanistan and Pakistan meet. It is the hub, the crow's nest, the fulcrum of Asia.
>
> —*John Keay*

The most exotic mountain valley ever associated with longevity is the one cut by the Hunza River amid the peaks of the Karakoram Range. Unlike the Caucasus or Vilcabamba, where tales of long-living people have historic roots, the Hunza claims are of recent vintage, their source traceable to the writings of a single individual: Sir Robert McCarrison. The background to his work was laid in the closing decades of the nineteenth century when the British extended the frontiers of their Indian empire into the western Himalayas. In a sustained effort that Rudyard Kipling called the Great Game, British agents, explorers, and adventurers sought to find passes leading into central Asia and to forge local military alliances for back-door challenges to the Russian and Chinese empires. As the decade of the 1890s opened, the last outpost in what is now Pakistan and was then the Northwest Frontier was the village of Gilgit. From that group of buildings, a narrow trail led into some of the most magnificent mountain grandeur available anywhere on earth. Mount Rakaposhi, the goddess of the snows, dominated the immediate vista, a peak of over 25,000 feet; and to the east was K-2, inferior in elevation only to Everest. Nestled among this splendor were minuscule robber states governed by autocratic despots called mirs. None was of more strategic importance than Hunza, a realm extending 50 miles east to west and 40 miles north to south.[1]

Given subsequent attempts to explain Hunzakut longevity partly as a function of a serene life-style amid idyllic surroundings, it is necessary to know something of the socioeconomic system prior to 1900. Politically, the state was ruled by the mir and his retinue of village chiefs. Their authority was absolute but unstable, as the mir's immediate relatives, backed by alternative village leaders, constantly plotted for power. Fratricide and patricide were frequent. Mir Mohammed Safdar Ali Khan, the ruler with whom the British negotiated in 1891, had gained his throne through murdering his father and at least one brother. Each successful revolt of this kind reshaped the pecking order in every village, unless the local headman had betrayed the former mir by shifting allegiances beforehand. Any losers in the power struggle who managed to escape with their lives retreated through the passes to neighboring states, where they spent most of their time trying to regain power.

Economically, Hunza's barely adequate agricultural output was dependent upon an excellent terrace and irrigation system engineered with a finesse that was the envy of surrounding peoples. But like their neighbors, the Hunzakuts could not have maintained their standard of living without collecting tribute from or raiding passing caravans. Independently or in alliance with others, the Hunzakuts would sweep out of their strongholds in periodic assaults on wealthy travelers. They could strike out at will and return to their valley, where various traps and fortifications made their villages impregnable. At times the road was just a series of rocks hammered into the side of the mountain. In an emergency, the rocks could be pulled loose, leaving a bare cliff face as Hunzakut warriors waited to start rockslides or use their weapons against any who dared venture farther. The value system was that of a typical warrior society in which, matters of politics aside, there was almost no crime within the society but in which pillage, rape, murder, and enslavement of outsiders were taken for granted.

The Hunzakuts claimed to be descended from stragglers in the army of Alexander the Great, namely three Greek soldiers and their Persian wives. Although nominally Moslem, their sect had some unorthodox practices. They drank a grape wine flavored with the oil of bitter apricots, their major crop; and it was customary until the 1930s for them to share their wives with respected visitors—a courtesy Europeans usually declined. Hunzakut women also went about unveiled and had more freedom than their sisters in other Islamic mirdoms. But the role of women was far from enviable. Free of physical mistreatment and permitted to do all the work men did except fighting, women were still considered congenitally stupid, and they were not allowed to travel alone, to be educated, or to own property. Males did not speak to females who were not in their families, and in Hunzakut homes there was only minimal communication between the sexes. The general contempt for women was so pronounced that as late as the 1950s outside observers noted that despondent women committed suicide by leaping from high ledges or by eating large quantities of apricot pits, which contain a substantial amount of cyanide. The possible emergence of an ebullient female on the order of Khfaf Lazuria or Kamachich Kvichenya was impossible.

Sexist values governed the treatment of domesticated animals as well. When winter approached, instead of reducing sheep herds by cutting them down to a majority of the sturdiest ewes and a few of the best rams, as is done in most cultures, the Hunzakuts maintained their herds at nearly full strength with an equal number of ewes and rams. This method placed an unnecessary strain on the limited vegetation and made a rapid spring buildup in the number of lambs improbable. Likewise, the Hunzakuts preferred stallions to mares even if the mares were hardier, on the assumption that in the long run the male of the species is always stronger. Rarely has male chauvinism taken such an awesome toll on the available food supply and immediate well-being of a people.

Old age was not honored either. McCarrison himself was shocked when the mirs throughout the Gilgit region could not understand why he wanted to "waste" medicine and other medical treatment on their aged.[2] One mir suggested that it would be a better idea to invent a lethal chamber to do away with the old quickly. As it was, many tribes required, upon pain of death, that the eldest son use a conical basket to carry his old and decrepit parents to a summit, where he was to drop them to their deaths. Similarly, after the major battles of the winter of 1891, old men were sent to deal with the British victors because it was feared envoys might be shot on sight and the old were deemed expendable. Except for a Council of Elders, whose members were appointed by the mir and could be dismissed at his pleasure, in traditional Hunza there were no social structures supportive of old age.

Until the war of 1891, the Mir of Hunza was contemptuous of all outsiders. The British were considered just one more warlike tribe of the kind that periodically rode up from Kashmir. When British demands became overbearing, the Mir would shout that his Chinese allies would send troops, or he would refer to his conversation with Captain Grombtchevski, the Russian explorer who had brought a Cossack troop through the northern passes with an offer of an alliance with the Tsar. In all these intrigues, the Mir sought to trade temporary concessions to any given foreign power for weapons and money. Eventually he overplayed his hand, and with Pathan troops, under British officers, playing a decisive role, he was militarily defeated and fled to exile in Sinkiang.

Mohammed Nazim Khan, a brother of the deposed mir,

agreed to accept British policy and became the new ruler of Hunza.[3] He was to prove a shrewd leader, and except for an end to the caravan raids, Hunzakut life under his reign and that of his successors, Ghazan Khan (1938–45) and Jamal Khan (1945–74), remained virtually unchanged. Of importance to the longevity tale about to unfold is the fact that the British military post remained at Gilgit, 60 miles from a semiautonomous Hunza.

During the 1890s, Robert McCarrison had been completing his medical studies at Oxford University. In 1901, at the age of 23, he sailed for India, where in 1902 he became a regimental officer in the Foreign Department. He quickly distinguished himself by correctly identifying a sand fly as the carrier of the Three Day Fever of Citral. Then, in 1904, McCarrison was appointed army surgeon to the nine villages of the Gilgit Agency, a post in which he was to serve until 1911. Shortly after his promotion, the young scientist began to do research on the goiter disease endemic throughout the agency. Finding eight villages afflicted with goiter and one free of it, McCarrison was able to discover the link to iodine deficiency. While traveling about in the area and making various health studies, McCarrison also came to certain conclusions about the health and longevity of the neighboring Hunzakuts. In the decades that followed his ideas on nutrition were to win him worldwide renown, and his writing on the Hunzakuts became so influential that by the 1970s no serious discussion of longevity around the world was complete without some reference to the remote Himalayan mirdom.

Robert McCarrison's claims for Hunza were threefold. The most important for him was that Hunzakuts were relatively free of many common diseases, especially those involving the gastrointestinal tract. Ailments like goiter and cretinism, scourges of Hunza's neighbors, were also said to be rare or unknown. McCarrison further stated that the Hunzakuts were long-living and that their incredible vigor persisted even at advanced ages. He related this splendid health profile to the quality of their diet. A summary view of Hunza appeared in *Studies in Deficiency Diseases*, written in 1921:

> My own experience provides an example of a race unsurpassed in perfection of physique and in freedom from disease in general, whose sole food consists to this day of grains, vegetables and fruit with a certain amount of milk and butter, and goat's meat only on feast days. I refer to the people of the state of Hunza, situated in the extreme northernmost point of India. . . . When the severe nature of the winter in that part of the Himalayas is considered, and the fact that their housing accommodations and conservancy arrangements are of the most primitive, it becomes obvious that the enforced restriction to the unsophisticated foodstuffs of nature is compatible with long life, continued vigor, and perfect physique.[4]

In 1938, McCarrison's views were given a more popular treatment in G. T. Wrench's well-written *The Wheel of Health*.[5] Never having been to India himself, Wrench quoted McCarrison extensively to establish the uniqueness of the Hunzakuts and then augmented McCarrison's claims with corroborating material from the writings of explorers and soldiers. For Wrench, as for McCarrison, Hunza was a land where the dietary habits and life-style he thought ideal had been tested successfully in nature's own laboratory. This view was buttressed by medical studies and presented in a manner that studiously avoided sensationalism. Over the years, Wrench's book became a standard reference on Hunza, referred to by other authors more frequently then McCarrison's own comments, which were scattered in his various essays written for a professional audience.

American exposure to Hunza got into high gear after 1949 with the publication of *The Healthy Hunzas* by J. I. Rodale, founder of the press that was to publish Grace Halsell's Vilcabamba book in 1976.[6] Like Wrench, Rodale had never been to India, and his views were based almost exclusively on the claims of McCarrison, again fleshed out

with a few supportive quotations from other sources. He
differed from Wrench by using language that was anything
but moderate; and his views were to be restated in increasingly flamboyant exaggerations by subsequent health
writers.

After the well-publicized trips of Lowell Thomas into the
Himalayas in the 1950s, a new thread in the Hunza cloth
began to be woven by such persons as a Nebraska optome-
trist, George Banik, who made a trip to Hunza under the
sponsorship of the *People Are Funny* television show, and Jay
Hoffman, a health lecturer seeking confirmation of his
favorite theories. The quality of the observations of such
travelers ran from amateurish to foolish. Jay Hoffman was to
call Hunza a Fountain of Youth where people frequently lived
to be well over 100.[7] His enthusiasm was exceeded by an
author in *The American Mercury*, who wrote, "No Hunzakut
has ever suffered from indigestion, constipation, ulcers,
cancer, or any venereal disease."[8] When told that some
Hunzakuts had lived to be 120 and even 140, Hoffman and
Banik cheerfully passed along the claims without asking for
any proof.[9] The champion of the faddist commentators was
Renée Taylor, who wrote or coauthored five books dealing
with life in Hunza.

The mythologizing of Hunza was also stimulated by the
1930s best seller *Lost Horizon*, which spawned successful
film, stage, radio, and television adaptations. In this popular
romance, James Hilton wrote of Shangri-La, a valley found
high in the Himalayas. Access was along a treacherous ice-
laden path open only for limited times of the year, but within
Shangri-La itself the climate was perfect. People entering
from the outside world found that the aging process was
slowed so that it took many decades to register the slightest
signs of wear. Led by a European priest, the outsiders
eventually formed a lamahood whose mission was to preserve human knowledge through the holocaust of wars the
twentieth century was doomed to endure. While not quite
pacifists in the Gandhian sense, the men and women of the

lamahood prized wisdom and virtue above all else. As the high lama explained, "We govern with moderate authority and we are pleased with moderate obedience."[10] This attitude and other characteristics of the fictional Shangri-La slowly attached to Hunza, which was usually depicted as almost inaccessible.

But Hunza, supposedly untouched since the march of Alexander, was actually a hub of international communications and espionage. During the latter part of the nineteenth century, the British had discovered that the other passes to Hunza were easier than the Gilgit route and that many travelers from Central Asia were accustomed to using Hunza as one of the passageways to India. The ill-defined frontier of Afghanistan was only 10 miles away, and the Russian tsar wished to push his empire to the Hunza border.

The writings of British agents who explored Hunza in the nineteenth century provide a fund of information about the society any centenarian surviving into the 1960s and '70s would have been born into. There are also accounts by various mountaineers, who, although usually more intrigued by glaciers than by human beings, sometimes dropped interesting asides on culture in their diaries. In 1934, Col. David Lorimer, who had served as the British agent in Gilgit from 1920 to 1924, commenced a fifteen-month stay in Hunza for the purpose of studying the native language. His wife wrote a detailed memoir of their experiences: the first year-round observation and the first substantial account of Hunzakut society.[11]

The decade of the '40s was to bring a flurry of visitors. Among the most unusual were a quartet of Norwegians who made a spectacular trip from Sweden through the Soviet Union into Hunza in an ostensible effort to join British forces in India for transport to an air school in Canada. The journal published by one of them appears somewhat naive, but the communication links cited are extremely sophisticated, and many native leaders thought the Great Game had entered a new phase.[12] In 1944 John Clark became active in Chinese

Turkestan as a reconnaissance engineer for General Joseph Stilwell, and from 1948 to 1951 he was in Hunza on various occasions. Clark was to write the most comprehensive and perceptive account of Hunza.[13] At about the same period as Clark's activities, the American journalists Jean and Frank Shor sought to retrace Marco Polo's journey. Their adventures included easy access to the Shah of Iran, a brush with the newly established Communist regime in China, and a stay in Hunza. They made a second trip to Hunza in 1952.[14] A few years later, Barbara Mons, a British woman inspired by reading Wrench and Lorimer, made a pilgrimage to Hunza, and in 1973 would come Alexander Leaf on the final leg of his longevity pilgrimage. In addition to these major commentators there were mountaineers, health teams, food faddists, hunters, and curiosity seekers of every description. Thus, there is a century-long continuum of information on Hunza against which McCarrison's thesis on Hunzakuts health may be evaluated.

At the core of McCarrison's assertions was the absence of certain common ailments among the Hunzakuts he treated. In his Mellon Lecture of 1921, McCarrison reported, "During my association with these people, I never saw a case of asthenic dyspepsia, of gastro or duodenal ulcer, or appendicitis. . . . While I cannot aver that all the maladies were quite unknown, I have the strongest reasons for the assertion that they were remarkably infrequent."[16] In *Studies in Deficiency Diseases*, published that same year, the point was put more boldly: "Such service as I was able to render them during the seven years I spent in their midst was confined chiefly to the treatments of accidental lesions, the removal of senile cataracts, plastic operations for granular lids, or the treatment of maladies wholly unconnected with the food supply. Appendicitis, so common in Europe, was unknown."[17] Later writings were to claim that Hunzakuts were free of cancer, heart disease, goiter, and cretinism.[18] What most intrigued McCarrison was the nature of the diet, to which he attributed the virtual immunity of Hunzakuts to gastrointestinal diseases.

On the issue of the Hunzakuts' overall health and the superiority of their natural diet, McCarrison and his followers were spectacularly off base. The most persistent thread in the Hunza commentary, from the first notes by Dr. G. W. Leitner[19] and Major Bidulph[20] in the 1860s and '80s to the most recent governmental reports, is the insufficiency of the food supply. In spite of the marvelous terraces carved on slopes as steep as 60 degrees, the amount of land available for cultivation is so meager and the arid soil so poor that not enough food can be grown to sustain the population. By the late spring of each year the food reserves run out, bringing on what is called Starvation Springtime. A pattern of two or three meals a week is common during this time. The Hunzakuts become so undernourished that vitamin-deficiency diseases cause ugly sores to appear on their bodies. Subclinical rickets and scurvy occur. If the winter is overly long or the first harvest poor, the effect is calamitous. Only massive outmigration has kept the valley from periodic famines. That McCarrison, a pioneer in understanding the centrality of vitamins and minerals to good health, should have chosen Hunza as an example of good diet is ironic. It would have served better as a warning of what happens when there are vitamin and mineral deficiencies. Indeed, if the Hunzakuts were as healthy as McCarrison believed, then the whole relationship of quality diet to good health would be called into question. However, the Hunzakuts are far from healthy.

The most devastating evidence about diseases in Hunza is found in the work of John Clark. Clark, as stated earlier, spent long periods of time in Hunza during every season, and he was one of the few Westerners to live independently of the Mir's largess. His interest in Hunza was partly based on his conviction that a modestly funded self-help program could create viable mountain economies that would be hostile to the central planning of the Communist regimes in China and the Soviet Union. To pursue his idea, Clark, a vertebrate paleontologist who was on the staff of the Chicago Museum of Natural History for many years, arrived in Hunza in 1950 with over a ton and a half of equipment and medicine. He had secured the cooperation of the Pakistan government by agreeing to make a free geological survey beyond that government's technical means, and he had obtained the Mir's lukewarm acceptance by pledging to open a dispensary. Nevertheless, regional officials in Gilgit accused him of being an American spy and plotted against him. Many of the older Hunzakuts who resented the modern ideas Clark spread among their youth complained to him and to the Mir. In addition to the geological survey and dispensary, Clark opened a handicraft school for boys, planted three experimental gardens, and taught all who would listen about new seeds he was prepared to give away. His plans were so thorough that he even brought along butterfly nets to collect specimens for the Carnegie Collection of High Altitude Butterflies. The work was to be done by Hunzakut boys who would be paid for their efforts.

The Hunza that Clark came to know bore little resemblance to the Shangri-La depicted by Wrench and Rodale. From the first day, his dispensary was mobbed by the ailing. Although the facility was open only on an irregular basis, Clark eventually treated 5,685 patients, or roughly one-fourth of the entire population. A great many of those he saw suffered from vitamin deficiencies or had stomach problems. Among the most common diseases were chronic dysentery, cataracts, malaria, impetigo, ringworm, trachoma, pneumonia, and some cases of tuberculosis.[21] Clark found that many Hunzakuts suffered from gastrointestinal pains, which he believed were due to the bitter apricot nut they used to flavor their wine. Malaria and dysentery reached epidemic proportions at various periods while he was in Hunza, and diseases were not confined to any one class. The royal family commandeered nearly a quarter of all medical supplies, particularly stomach remedies, and they would have taken more if he had not resisted their demands. Whenever Clark undertook local trips, he discovered that the Mir would spread word of his coming by telephone so that people from some of the outer villages could consult him for medical treatment.

Wrench had written that Hunza's vegetables were "much like ours,"[22] yet among the new crops introduced by Clark in 1950 were beets, lettuce, endive, radishes, turnips, spinach, yellow pear tomatoes, Brussels sprouts, and parsley: the heart of the Anglo-American garden. Clark also noted that the apricot trees had reddish leaves at the growing tips, a sign of soil deficiency. He found that manure was not plentiful and except for human waste had to be laboriously brought down from the heights where there were goats and sheep. There was so little Vitamin D in the diet that calcium was difficult to assimilate. This caused the teeth of the Hunzakuts to be extremely soft and loose. Clark developed beriberi during his first winter there and thought the whole population had a deficiency of Vitamin A, Vitamin D, and the Vitamin B complex.

Support for Clark's observations was provided later in the decade by Barbara Mons, whose agenda included an inquiry into Hunzakut diseases. To that end she questioned Dr. Safdar Mahmood of the Pakistan Medical Corps, who had established a clinic in Hunza. Dr. Mahmood showed her how the light in his operating room was adjusted for the numerous appendectomies he performed. In 1958, he said, he had treated 348 cases of dysentery, 1 case of typhoid, 734 cases of intestinal disease, 290 malaria cases, 113 cases of rheumatic fever, and 426 goiters for a total of more than 1,900 cases in a population of from 26,000 to 30,000 persons.[23] Mons reported that spring was still a most difficult time of the year, but that the potatoes introduced by the British had helped stave off starvation.

Fifteen years after the Mons visit, the trail from Gilgit was being transformed into a military road to enable China to reinforce Pakistan in case of war with India. Using the new artery in the making was Alexander Leaf, who found health conditions in Hunza not much better than those observed by Mons and Clark. Dr. Sahoor Ahmed, who had volunteered to serve as a medical doctor in Hunza to fulfill his required two years of military duty, had been at his post for eight months when Leaf arrived. Dr. Ahmed reported that there were now eight dispensaries and one hospital in Hunza, with the dispensaries staffed by nonphysicians. Hunzakuts didn't like to remain in the hospital, but their health was not good. Infant mortality was higher than in Punjab, and diarrheal disorders were the major cause. Leaf summarized Ahmed's views as follows:

> [Ahmed] found malnutrition, anemia, worms, goiter with many cretins, and pneumonia to be common. There was a smallpox outbreak with three or four deaths in the past year. . . . Tuberculosis is found among the young males who go "down country" for military service and employment in Pakistan, but women also have tuberculosis. There is much bronchial asthma. . . . Everyone, he claimed, had worms—round worms, tape worms, and thread worms.[24]

How is it possible to square the observations of Clark, Mons, Mahmood, and Ahmed with that of McCarrison and the food faddists? One answer is that most visitors to Hunza came when the weather had cleared and the valley was in full bloom. By this time, many symptoms of malnutrition had been cured or ameliorated by the first harvest. In addition, visitors were usually guests of the Mir and were not very knowledgeable in the local language or Asian culture. Understandably, the Mir, seeking good publicity for his realm, was not about to show his sick and lame or to talk about the perennial threat of famine. One might argue that the pre-1940 Hunza was more prosperous, but this is contradicted by repeated observations from the earliest visitors about the inadequate food supply and the fact that new crops and medicines introduced by the Europeans had been helpful. But

McCarrison had spent seven full years at the Gilgit Agency. Surely he knew Hunza better than those who stayed even as long as two years.

Perhaps not. It is possible that McCarrison's visits were limited to the summer season or that he never actually set foot in Hunza proper at all! McCarrison's station was Gilgit; he would not have gone to Hunza at the end of the summer for fear of getting snowed in, and he would not have gone immediately at the end of winter because of the dangerous trail. His writings give no indication that he ever saw the cycle of seasons as Clark and the Lorimers did. It is noticeable, too, that while McCarrison comments on the precarious nature of the food supply, he does not mention the diseases of malnutrition that his physician's eye would have spotted at once. It is also extremely suspicious that in his writings about the Hunzakuts he is coy about naming them, usually referring to "peoples of the Himalayan foothills." In one essay, McCarrison stated that his Hunzakut patients came 60 miles to be treated: the exact distance between Gilgit and Hunza.[25] There is every likelihood that the majority of Hunzakuts he treated, perhaps the only ones, were soldiers of the Hunza Rifles, the finest specimens of Hunzakut manhood. This interpretation is strengthened by his admission that he never treated a female. Other sources indicate that the Hunzakuts did not shield their women from outsiders, and even though it was forty years later, Clark, Mahmood, and Ahmed all treated female patients. With the exception of the royal entourage, women were not allowed to travel and could not venture as far as Gilgit. The mirs, in fact, restricted all travel unless it was for a permanent move or in their service. Only the most unusual circumstances would have brought the seriously ill, the old, and children to Gilgit.

McCarrison's terminology is not very satisfactory either. References to Indian peoples habitually mix caste, religious, and ethnic classifications. His often-used phrase "the fighting races of India" takes in Pathans, Sikhs, Punjabis, Dogras, Rajputs, Brahmins, and Jats. He wrote, "Among these, the

Sikhs, the Pathans, and certain Himalayan tribes, one cannot find whether in the East or West, finer physical development, hardihood, and powers of energy."[26] He credits these attributes to diet. The Sikhs favored food with a root base and the Pathans cereal, while the Hunzakuts had a combination of both. Other McCarrison essays were to compare Hunzakuts to tribes of the Nile and the west coast of Africa. None of these African or Asian groups has ever been cited for long life or immunity to disease. The impression is strong that McCarrison imbued the Hunzakuts with the benefits of his perfect diet without closely examining their lives or their general health. He was to be in India many times after his 1904–11 tour of duty, but he never again visited Hunza, and in his collected writings, published in 1972, no work dealing with Hunza is included. Nor did McCarrison ever write an essay in which the Hunzakuts were the major topic. All this seems odd treatment for a people he had identified early in his distinguished career as the living confirmation of his basic theories.

Except for McCarrison, none of the on-site writers before the 1950s mentions extraordinary longevity in Hunza, or large numbers of older inhabitants, much less supercentenarians. Rudyard Kipling, who used every legend he could when writing about India, did not touch on longevity legends when utilizing Hunza as one of the models for episodes in *Kim* and *The Man Who Would Be King*. At best, the historical record contains an occasional reference to an individual's being old, without a specific age cited. The Lorimers, when told one man was a centenarian, thought him to be in his 90s, and they described a woman of 50 as "a beautiful old woman."[27] At the handicraft school, Clark found that his boys and their parents had only an approximate sense of their age. One boy jumped in age from 13 to 17 in less than two full years. Clark concluded, "There is no evidence that anyone ever reached one hundred years of age in Hunza."[28] Mons supplemented this view by commenting, "That they are abnormally long lived is impossible to prove for the simple reason that no record is kept of a child's birth. They do not know how old they are."[29]

It must be stated in McCarrison's behalf that when he first went to Gilgit, the average life-span in the Kashmir Valley was in the early twenties. People in their 50s were considered old, and one reputed to be in his 90s was thought a wonder.[30] By this standard, if Hunzakuts were reaching their 70s and 80s in any number, they might well be thought of as long-living. Likewise, while Hunzakut infant mortality rates might be much higher than those in the developed world, they have always compared well with those of Kashmir. By taking McCarrison's comments out of their historical context, popularizers may have seriously distorted his original intent. In any case, his claims were never expressed in numbers but only in generalities.

Among the few visitors to give specific ages of Hunzakuts were the Shors. They wrote that the 12-man Council of Elders had one 97-year-old representative, while the rest were in their 70s and 80s. At social events, the Shors found other men who claimed to be nonagenarians even though they were not members of the Council. They do not report on any centenarians. At about the time of their first visit, the Mir had received an inquiry from J. Rodale concerning Hunzakut life-spans. The Mir responded in a letter dated August 24, 1947, that barring accidents, most of his people lived at least into their mid-80s.[31] A few years later, after the Mir had visited the West, he was telling visitors like Banik and Hoffman that some of his subjects had lived to 120 and an isolated few to 140—a rather spectacular revision. By the time Leaf came on the scene, the maximum age cited by the Mir was under 110. Only a few centenarians were available for actual examination at that time, but Leaf was assured that previous generations had been healthier, happier, and longer-lived. The only attempt at a proof of old age was the statement of one man that when he was in his 20s he had served in the War of 1891 as one of the Mir's bodyguards.

Women are noticeably absent from Hunzakut longevity

claims. Apparently, like the Hunzakut ewes and mares, they are not as strong as the male of the species, an exception to the worldwide rule. Also absent are multigenerational families. Since Hunzakuts often marry while in their teens, if many people were living into their 90s, five-generation families should be available. This would certainly be true if, as later claimed by the Mir, there were scores of centenarians alive in the 1940s and '50s. Yet Leaf saw only four-generational families, and Clark, while told of five-generational families, also saw only four generations among Hunzakuts he knew well. Clark made the further point that since the poor mineral content of the food produced extremely soft and loose teeth, a genuine Hunzakut centenarian would likely have all of his or her teeth ground to the gums. He had never seen such a Hunzakut. His own evaluation was that because of the terrible hardships of mountain life, those who succeeded in living past 60 were good septuagenarian and octogenarian bets, but that only a few survived much of their tenth decade. Such a pattern would be consistent with other mountain regions in developing nations.

All that remains of McCarrison's vision is the strong physique of the Hunzakuts. Here he is on unassailable ground. The strength, agility, and hardiness of the Hunzakuts has been remarked on by every visitor. One veteran mountaineer considered them "the world's best slab climbers."[32] Another saw a man dive into an ice-filled river.[33] Several observed that Hunzakuts could travel over Himalayan terrain at the rate of more than 40 miles a day.[34] Other examples of endurance lace every Hunza diary or book. The overall strength of the Hunzakuts has been confirmed in repeated medical tests as well. Of great interest to gerontologists is that Hunzakuts have almost no cancer or cardiovascular disease, providing one more instance in which the so-called degenerative diseases are not found among the old or middle-aged.

The toughness of the Hunzakuts can be misunderstood if it is taken out of the context of Himalayan culture and their physiques are compared with the flabby bodies typical of sedentary cultures. Many of the explorers who extolled the virtues of the Hunzakuts made equally flattering comments about Pathans and Sherpas. Faddist writers who quote them overlook this, giving the impression that the Hunzakuts were considered a unique biological elite. Racist overtones also creep into much Hunza commentary. The Hunzakuts are described as being lighter-skinned and taller than their neighbors, as if these were attributes of health. Some of the most balanced judgments came from the British military. The legendary Colonel Younghusband wrote:

> . . . they [the Hunzakuts] were capable of marching 40 miles in the day armed and equipped across the mountains. And they had an extraordinary elan and capacity for working rapidly under their own leaders. In Chital, Yasin, and other little states on the frontier, *I subsequently found the same thing.* [Emphasis added].[35]

Generally when there is a sustained comparison of Hunzakuts with other Himalayans, it is with their nearest neighbors, the Nagirs, who live on the opposite side of the Hunza River. In 1893 the British staged sports contests, and the Hunzakuts emerged victorious every time. Most subsequent writing refers to their continuing physical superiority to the Nagirs. The Hunzakuts are said to be neat, friendly, and hygienic, while the Nagirs are described as slovenly, surly, and dirty. The Hunzakuts also are praised for being better agriculturalists, engineers, hunters, and soldiers. While there may be an element of truth in these dichotomies, the qualities mentioned often focus on just those areas most favorable to the Hunzakuts and prove much less than the authors believe. Much too much has certainly been made of the belief that the two groups had a common ancestor and that they are separated only by a single river. The shorter and darker cast of the Nagir physical type comes from frequent intermarriage with the people of the Kashmir Valley, who have influenced Nagir in numerous ways. And the Hunza

River is no cute mountain stream. For centuries it was traversed by a narrow rope bridge which collapsed several times every summer. As a cultural barrier it was every bit as formidable as the Great Wall of China.

Of possible health significance is the extraordinary personal hygiene of the Hunzakuts which is in marked contrast to all the surrounding peoples. This could have had a positive effect, particularly during the time when infectious diseases, unchecked by modern drugs, were the most common threat to health. Even this virtue, however, may have been overstressed or confused by subjective value judgments. Too often, slovenly dress simply means clothing styles unlike those seen in Europe. Pioneers in colonial America erroneously believed native Americans to be slovenly and dirty because of the skins, feathers, tattoos, and jewelry the native Americans favored. The situation was aggravated during times of conflict, when the native Americans used war paint and other techniques to horrify their opponents.

Another factor not fully appreciated by native travelers was the rivalry between Hunza and Nagir. If one journeyed to Hunza first and became friendly with its mir, the welcome across the river was not likely to be cordial. The British officers who happened to befriend the Nagirs first usually preferred them to the Hunzakuts, believing them to be quicker learners and to possess a more democratic temperament. The military certainly was not impressed by the bravery or skills of the Hunzakut fighters. After losing the major battles of 1891, the Hunzakuts had not waged a guerrilla war but had meekly accepted the new mir's authority. The only reason they had ever been the senior partners in the Nagir-Hunza alliance was their geographic situation. Nagir was in a cul-de-sac, which made it more vulnerable to a prolonged siege or to a frontal assault than Hunza was. Military diarists observed other significant terrain factors. Hunza faced south and got far more sunlight than Nagir. During two months of the year, some villages in Nagir could count the daily sunlight in minutes if they got any sun at all. The effects on the growing season, crop quality, and individual dispositions are obvious.

The Hunza Council of Elders is another topic variously interpreted. The faddists have tried to liken it to a democratic or people's court of venerables. Such a view sadly underestimates the absolute authority of the mir. Early in the British contact, when Younghusband was showing a new rifle to a mir, he was told to fire at a man across the valley. Younghusband objected and the Mir became incensed, stating that the target was his man and had no more rights than his goats or sheep.[36] The shrewdest evaluation of the Mir's council was made by Clark. He saw that rather than holding office by virtue of age or as representatives of their local villages, the council members were appointees of the Mir. Clark witnessed overnight changes in the council when the Mir became displeased. This sort of arrangement has little relation to Western concepts of parliament or even a jury of peers. The daily convening of the council was more akin to the practice in Saudi Arabia, where even the humblest subject may come to court to present a direct appeal to the ruling aristocracy. The justice obtained may be swift, fair, and humane, but it is linked to the notion of the divine right of sovereigns. With no independent political, social, or economic base, the Council of Elders had no power to check the mir's authority.

The policy of the mirs from 1892 to 1974 was consistent. They hoped to hold on to their power by keeping the population as insulated from outside influence as possible. The Hunza Rifles were disbanded at the first opportunity, and with varying success, the mirs discouraged the idea of their young men being eligible for military duty "down country." Travel that did not result in permanent migration was discouraged, and foreign visitors were monitored with care. The telephones installed by the British and shortwave radios were handled in a way that strengthened the mirs' control rather than opening Hunza to wider cross-cultural contacts.

For more than eighty years, the mirs maneuvered

adroitly between contending foreign and regional powers. When the Hindu leadership in Kashmir decided to align that state with India even though the population was predominantly Moslem, the Mir withdrew Hunza from Kashmir to become part of Islamic Pakistan. In 1971, he explained to Leaf that he had been successful in combating corrosive outside influences, especially among "the students" who were restless.[37] Early in 1974, when informed that the Pakistan government intended to terminate Hunza's autonomy, the Mir said the people supported him overwhelmingly and would revolt if he were displaced. But that September, nine hundred years of autonomous and sometimes benevolent feudalism came to an end with the support of most of the Hunzakuts. Although the Mir was stripped of his secular power, he was allowed to continue to serve as a representative of the Aga Khan and was given a princely pension and a lowland palace. To the end, the man who had done so much to promote the myth of Hunzakut longevity continued to play the Shangri-La game. He told reporters of the international press that while there were only 5 or 6 centenarians presently alive, before the work on the military road had begun in 1958 there had been 50 to 60.[38] He did not explain why Mons, the Shors, Clark, the Lorimers, and so many others had never seen them. By 1979, when the Karakoram Highway was formally opened, the Mir had died, but his 36-year-old son and successor, Ghazanfar Ali, was still fielding queries about supercentenarians. "No, no, not 120 and 130 years. But we do have a lot of people between 90 and 100 years old," he replied. The reasons given for such ages were "good, pure food, peace, freedom from stress, and no crime."[39]

It is amazing that the myth of Hunzakut longevity has persisted for such a long time on such flimsy evidence. Hunza was never significantly different from dozens of other tiny Himalayan mirdoms. Since the first British contacts in the nineteenth century, the specifics have altered, but not the patterns of internal life and foreign contacts. The Dowager Empress and the Tsar have been replaced by feuding commissars. The British influence has given way to that of the United States. Territorial and religious rivalries have created the states of Pakistan and India, still squabbling with each other and with Afghanistani and Kashmiri politicians about viable frontiers. Meanwhile, the old trade route coming down from Central Asia has become the Karakoram Highway, with the little huts once maintained by the mir for travelers replaced by hotels and camping grounds able to accommodate 12,000 annual visitors.

The Hunza myth demonstrates anew that however depressing the human record may be, the species wants to believe that somewhere on earth it has managed to produce a society where war, crime, poverty, injustice, and disease have been abolished. For almost a hundred years, the Anglo-American world has thought it was a tiny kingdom just beyond the last imperial outpost. Perhaps with improved food supplies and adequate medical services coupled with more social opportunities for women and the young, Hunza may yet experience a longevity boom. But Hunza never had a golden age, and Hunza was never Shangri-La. The only Valley of the Blue Moon is in the fiction of James Hilton, and unless they are in the entourage of the Abominable Snowman, there are no supercentenarians in the Himalayas.

6

SERENDIPITOUS SHERINGHAM AND CAMBRIDGESHIRE

> I was born in a garden, and I have
> been in one ever since.
>
> —*James Chapman, age 103*

Gerontologists who had been wary of longevity stories emanating from isolated and distant regions of the world were startled in the early 1970s when a village only 125 miles from London was thrust into the longevity spotlight.[1] David Davies, one of the advocates of the Vilcabamba claims, had discovered that in Upper Sheringham the number of inhabitants over age 60 was more than triple the national British average. The population of approximately 300 contained a number of nonagenarians and a vigorous centenarian. Davies' analysis of the Sheringham soil had shown that it was unusually rich in minerals, particularly selenium, identified previously as a possible prolongevous substance. As almost every villager ate vegetables grown in the local gardens and greenhouses, the tentative linkage of a mineral-rich soil and long life showed promise.

Proceeding on these few facts, journalists and television

reporters from several nations descended on the quiet Norfolk village, which seemed to have endured from another and better era. Its houses, built with a gray sea stone in styles that blend into the natural landscape as if planned by a consummate architect, caught the attention of many of the photojournalists. Others took haunting shots of All Saints Church, built in the 1300s, and made appropriate close-ups of the graveyard stones marking the life-spans of deceased longevous villagers. Still others favored the Red Lion Pub, which still served a gigantic "Ploughman's Share" luncheon. If serenity and beauty were Methuselah factors, then Upper Sheringham was a Britannic Shangri-La.

Apparently the aesthetics of Upper Sheringham were so powerful that they lulled reporters into ignoring the normal investigative inquiries. Readily available census tables revealed that the Upper Sheringham statistics had been grossly misinterpreted.[2] While it was quite true that 18 percent of the Upper Sheringham population was over 60, compared with the national average of 5 percent and a regional average of 12 percent, it was also true that owing to economic factors, the entire northern coast was in demographic imbalance with the rest of the country. At the same time that the lovely shore, sloping hills, and relatively low cost of living had attracted an influx of retirees, economic stagnation had been driving out many younger people. In a 1978 interview, "Chick" Denis, an elected official of Sheringham proper, estimated that from 65 to 85 percent of the population was not native-born and that the age range of 25 to 45 had been decimated by the need to move elsewhere to find employment.[3]

The pattern Denis described was typical for the whole coast. Consulting the census figures for the 1970s, it is possible to determine that the population over 60 in areas surrounding Sheringham differs from it by only a few percentage points and that in some it exceeds the Sheringham figures. The same results obtain when the percentage of longevous people is calculated, again with some neighboring areas having a slightly higher and some a slightly lower number than Sheringham.[4] As the British census count is rounded off to the nearest 5, the variations are statistically insignificant.

The results for Upper Sheringham, a village separated from the main town by less than a mile, are further imbalanced by a retirees' home located at the edge of one of the approaches to the village. The Dales, a beautiful residence which once belonged to the vicar, generally houses about 30 persons over age 60. Its most famous occupant in the decade of the '70s was Frederick Cornelius, who had been born on January 14, 1874, in Dover and died on December 24, 1979, three weeks short of 106.[5] At 104, Cornelius was still taking buses and taxicabs unaided and liked to stroll the quarter-mile to the local post office. He conversed lucidly, telling visitors of his fighting days in India, when he had been a color sergeant in the Scottish Rifles. Enjoying his notoriety as one of the oldest men in Great Britain, Cornelius talked about awards from his old regiment, payments from his insurance company, telegrams from Queen Elizabeth, and similar events. Most mornings he would be up before six, bathing, shaving, and dressing himself before going out for a walk in the lovely garden adjacent to The Dales. The final phase of his morning routine was to take up a position under a broad-branched tree where he fed birds with a tranquil dignity that conjured up images of St. Francis of Assisi.

Charming as Frederick Cornelius might be, his longevity had little significance for the selenium theorists, as he was already in his late 90s before coming to The Dales, and unlike most others in the home, he had not even lived much of his life in any part of Norfolk. After his military service he had sold insurance and then been a greengrocer in Kent. In one of those ironies which make longevity research so fascinating, Cornelius was advised at age 49 to retire because of a heart ailment. The worried doctor had long since died, while Cornelius, though frail and sleeping away a goodly part of the day, could still handle his own affairs with considerable humor. Pointing to his ears, Cornelius would inform a visitor that his deafness made "a proper conversation difficult," but he knew what the visitor was interested in, so he would begin a discourse about his personal habits, eating preferences, and views of the world. Mrs. Musgrove, the director of The Dales, joked with him a great deal and would comment, "I think he's at a point where he only hears what he wishes to hear." In spite of press shots that showed him clutching a bottle of stout or holding a cigar, Cornelius did not drink alcohol in any form, had never smoked, and had been a light eater all his life. Until his final days he kept a watchful eye on his finances, flirted with the staff, and took pleasure in playing whist, checkers, and dominoes.

The Upper Sheringham hoax might be put to rest at this point except for the work of a remarkable local scholar, A. Campbell Erroll. After retiring from a banking firm in London, Erroll made a hobby of local history. His greatest service was the methodical tabulating of the registers of the local parishes. Gathering together every scrap of information available about the area, he published a history of Sheringham in 1970 and deposited research materials in the Norfolk Library in Norwich.[6]

Long before the longevity story became popular, Erroll had computed all the births, baptisms, and deaths recorded in Old Saints Church from 1789 through the mid-1860s. After 1868 the church records cease to be comprehensive, because of new churches in the area and dissent within the Church of England. Persons born in Upper Sheringham might be buried elsewhere, and vice versa, making the reconstruction of individual life-spans difficult or impossible. During the early periods, however, one is able to follow most persons from the cradle to the grave with some knowledge of the kind of work they did and which part of the area they lived in. Not the least of Erroll's contributions is to point out that the persons buried in Old Saints include not only the inhabitants of

Upper Sheringham, but those of the town as well, people who generally obtained their vegetables from the same sources as the rest of Norfolk.

A study within the wider Sheringham project was Erroll's attempt to re-create the life of the village from 1791 to 1838. Out of a population of about 350 persons, Erroll found that most of the population were agricultural workers and fishermen, followed by craftspeople and mechanics. There were also a handful of merchants, 1 schoolmaster, 1 vicar, and 1 gentleman. Then Erroll made a fascinating discovery: "It may be significant to note that of the 206 persons whose age at death is known, seven attained the age of 90 or more, forty-four were 80 or over, and one hundred and six were over 70."[7] These figures work out to at least 30 percent of the population's living to an age greater than 70. Making a further breakdown, Erroll was able to determine that there were no significant differences in life-span between those residing in Upper Sheringham and those in the town.

Erroll had stumbled upon a kind of two-tier longevity profile, which is confirmed by an even casual perusal of the church registers. Throughout most of the nineteenth century, those who did not die as infants or children had a very good probability of living past 60. Page after page of the registers, written in the neat script of various vicars, show that deaths occurred mainly either under the age of 20 or after 60.[8] From 1813 to 1857, out of 800 burials there are 66 septuagenarians, 63 octogenarians, and 9 nonagenarians. From 1858 to 1921, there are 1,600 burials, with 381 septuagenarians, 160 octogenarians, and 30 nonagenarians. Both time periods work out to about 18 percent of the total population's living over seventy years. Even accounting for the fact that after the mid-1800s the records do not give a comprehensive picture of the area's population, there is the strongest suggestion that Sheringham, while not having phenomenal longevity, has been an area where life-spans have constantly been at the upper levels of normal. The oldest recorded age at death before 1960 was 98.

In follow-up work covering the period 1960–78, Erroll has consulted the burial records for the six major religious institutions in the district. While the significance of the number of persons dying at advanced ages cannot be determined because of the tremendous inmigration of retirees, it is interesting to note that in a period of eighteen years, there have been 74 deaths of persons over age 90, 9 of whom exceeded the longest life-span recorded in the preceding two centuries. There were 3 centenarians, 1 person who died four days short of 100, 2 persons over 99, and 3 over 98. At the very least these findings would indicate that the Sheringham environment is not hostile to long life.

Sheringham's history reveals that it has been a neglected rural area for more than three hundred years, primarily devoted to agriculture and fishing and with no large industries. The first post office was opened in 1856; the railroad arrived in 1887; the first bank was established in 1890, and the first county library was organized in 1928. Just as the longevity writers had stated, many residents of even modest means had greenhouses attached to their homes, making possible a year-round supply of fresh vegetables. A common planting ground in the center of the village was available to any inhabitant for cultivation, and older people unable to tend plots were given produce by those who could. Muck bins, a relative of the American compost heap, provided fertilizer. Although the Sheringham area has almost no snowfall and has one of the driest climates in England, it has a bracing atmosphere provided by prevailing winds blowing directly across the North Sea from regions of the Arctic.

Life in seaside Sheringham during the nineteenth century has been graphically reconstructed by Stanley Craske, another dedicated local historian. He has drawn extensively from stories told to him by grandparents, parents, and fisherfolk. Until mid-century, Upper Sheringham had been the undisputed center of gravity, where the gentry, vicar, and schoolmaster lived and entertained. On the shoreline were fishing families operating some two hundred fifty boats and earning a living from the sea. Constantly referred to as insolent rebels, the people of Lower Sheringham came to be called Shannocks, from the old English word *shanny* meaning "reckless" or "daredevil." The Shannocks asserted their independence by leaving the Church of England in great numbers to become Methodists or to enroll in the Salvation Army. One of the prides of the community was a lifeboat service established in 1838. When ships floundered in the North Sea, the Shannocks rowed out to save lives and to claim salvage rights.

The fisherfolk were extremely hardy, and like the Abkhasians, they never really retired. Men worked in the boats until their 70s and 80s and then mended nets and performed other shore work. Because the males went to sea during their early teens, the women had more formal education. As a consequence, in addition to traditional household duties, women managed the family finances and often instructed their husbands in reading and writing, thus deriving a stature not enjoyed by many working-class women of that era.

The strong-willed fishing clans account for many of the octogenarians and nonagenarians found in the Sheringham registers. Anecdotes about them recorded by Craske confirm what Thoms had written about the same name's running in a family. It is said that at one time in Sheringham there may have been as many as 16 men with the name John Henry Grice. They were differentiated by their nicknames. This same practice is found in the West family, in which fishermen of the same name were known as Spider West, Never Sweat West, Sugar West, Teapot West, and other endearing identifications.

Returning to contemporary Upper Sheringham, if people living at The Dales are excluded, in 1978 the oldest inhabitant was Rosie Runcieman, age 90, and the oldest native-born inhabitant was Reggie Chastney, age 83, whose family name is frequently found among the long lives recorded in Old Saints Church. Chastney relates that his parents and relatives used to tell him that it was typical for workers to walk both ways to farms 5 and 10 miles distant each day, an observation repeated by several persons knowledgeable about the area. Ivy Chastney, age 73, Reggie's wife, thought it might be important that the area had a tradition of homemade fruit wines and beer. It was the couple's opinion that people weren't living as long as they used to because life had gotten considerably softer.

While the Chastneys enjoyed speculating about longevity with visitors, their attitude was not shared by most of their neighbors, who were somewhat fearful that too much publicity would bring a flood of sight-seers. They were particularly turned off by the idea that those "dreadful California types" would besiege them. Many did not think that there was any more longevity in their village than elsewhere in Norfolk, and they pointed out that the tombstones bore witness to many short lives as well. Displaying the proverbial common sense of the British, they thought it sensible, not remarkable, that a gardener, age 72, should ride his bicycle while performing errands. "It's cheaper than petrol and invigorating," said one woman as she weeded her garden. Another similarity to Abkhasia was the church choir, which was made up entirely of pensioners.

A health advantage enjoyed by the people of the entire Norfolk coast which is far less mysterious than the properties of selenium is that they have been able to relish their pastoral cake without passing up the benefits of modern medicine. Easy access to medicines and treatment relating to minor diseases, which thereby are kept from developing into something more serious, are probably more important to longevity than spectacular surgery or other high-technology medicine. The people of Norfolk also share in the welfare state. The most obvious prolongevous expression of this is The Dales, which is part of a system operated by the Social Services department of the central government. Unlike hospitals and related institutions, The Dales belongs to a category of homes operated for seniors who need some assistance but can manage most of their daily tasks on their own. It provides only the most minimal medical assistance, being more like a government-run boardinghouse than a health institution. Meals and housekeeping are provided for residents, but if they wish, they may aid in both tasks. Half the residents at The Dales have private rooms, while the other half share their quarters. Roommates are chosen by the residents rather than being assigned by the director, and individuals ask to become residents rather than being assigned by an agency. The waiting lists are long, and health professionals feel that less than 10 percent of the population that would like the service is being accommodated. Frederick Cornelius stated bluntly that he would not have been able to enjoy as many birthdays as he had if he had not been able to live in a place like The Dales where he could be assisted when the need arose yet could preserve his autonomy.

Another home of the same variety is found in Overstrand, less than an hour's drive from Sheringham. Called Sea Marge, it was once owned by a German industrialist. Later the mansion served as a hotel for British dignitaries, including Winston Churchill, George Bernard Shaw, and King George V. Gracing one of the rooms of Sea Marge in 1978 was a huge photograph taken seven years earlier showing 11 women with a combined age of 1,039 years. The occasion was the celebration by 10 nonagenarians of the 100th birthday of Mrs. M. E. Cubitt. Robert Devenny, the director of Sea Marge, stated that the nonagenarian residents he had known through the years had lived rather ordinary lives before coming to Sea Marge and had no peculiar dietary or personal habits. Most had been agricultural workers, housewives, and domestics, but he thought this mainly reflected the need of the poor to take advantage of government services while the middle class and the rich made other provisions. Few of the nonagenarians he had known had ever consumed much alcohol or smoked at any time during their lives. Devenny emphasized that homes like The Dales and Sea Marge were unusual in that they had been converted from luxury housing. In most of the system, the homes were expressly constructed for older people, having such facilities as ramps and roomy elevators for getting to upper floors.

Orchard House, a low-slung modern edifice of the kind Devenny had in mind, is located in Sawston, a town just outside Cambridge in the direction of London. In 1978, it had a much more dynamic ambiance than either Sea Marge or The Dales. Although housing many permanent residents, it was also an active service center. Hot meals were prepared and taken to persons living at home, and many people used the facilities for various daytime social functions. One service that Brenda Tarrant, the director, thought was quite important in promoting longevity was that older people could live in the facility if the people they usually resided with wanted to take a vacation or were temporarily unable to care for them. Mrs. Tarrant was also pleased about another distinction of Orchard House: it was the home of 108-year-old Alice Empelton, the oldest woman in Great Britain.

Until the age of 106 Alice Empelton had lived by herself in a small bungalow, having an occasional meal brought in or getting assistance for heavier house chores. She expressed a strong desire to get back on her own if she could somehow regain her strength. In spite of poor hearing and frailty, Alice at 108 was alert and extremely congenial. After a whole morning's interview, instead of being tired, she said she felt invigorated. She enjoyed being with other people and didn't mind expressing her views. Far from harping on the "good old days," she felt there had been tremendous improvements since her birth in 1870, and she looked forward to more. Having been a victim of poverty, she had no love for the well-to-do:

> I'm Labor. Always was. I worked for them. I canvassed for them. Yes, I'm Labor. Staunch. So was my husband. He was for them too. I'd work for them again. You know, I saw Queen Victoria at her Diamond Jubilee in 1897. I was on my honeymoon. I thought she looked rather shabby for a queen. . . . When I was young, girls couldn't have a career. I

wanted to be a schoolteacher. I went through exams, but when
it came to the supplementary, I couldn't take it, because my
mother could not afford to support me for three more years.
There was no factory work then, so I had to get work as a
domestic. To this day I remember how I walked up the stairs
for two hours at a time every day hauling hot water for them.
There were only jugs and washstands in those days. You don't
know what a miracle a hot-water faucet is. You just can't
imagine. Another thing to remember is that we didn't have
help then. There was no unemployment benefits, no medical
assistance. We just suffered.

Alice went on to state that until her marriage at age 27, she
had never ceased to feel tired. Although she had never had
any children of her own, she had brought up 8, some of whom
she was still in contact with. "I didn't have time to darn my
stockings," she says without a hint of regret. In later life,
particularly after she became widowed in 1939, she spent a
lot of time in her flower and vegetable gardens as well as
remaining active in social causes. Alice had never had much
use for medicine and was not a big eater. "I've always liked
fruit. An orange a day is good to keep you going."

As the interview with Alice drew to a close, her reminiscing was interrupted by the entrance of a jaunty white-
haired woman walking with the aid of an aluminum frame.
The newcomer was Rachel Rennie, who could have been
taken for 74 as easily as for her actual 104. She had come to
report to Alice on newspaper and television coverage of
Alice's recent birthday party. Almost totally blind, Rachel
had a cheerful disposition and a blissful singsong cadence in
her voice. She quipped that she listened to rather than
watched the television program. The two centenarians had
met only recently, and Rachel was eager to know more about
her new friend's life. A temporary resident at Orchard House,
who would return to her daughter's home when her daughter
came back from a vacation, Rachel spoke little about her own
life other than to say that she had walked a great deal and
liked to exercise. Asked her reaction to Orchard House, she

thought it was "a bit quiet" and was anxious to get home. "It's unsettling to be away from your things."

Conversations with Brenda Tarrant and Norman Tarrant, her deputy and husband, revealed that there was a third centenarian living at Orchard House: Flo Evans, age 100. Unfortunately, Mrs. Evans was too ill to see visitors. The Tarrants knew of several other centenarians living in Cambridgeshire. One of their favorites was Mrs. Florence Jeaps, age 104, a lively conversationalist. Another was Mrs. Polly Wilson, age also 104, who had had a sweet pea named in her honor by the W. J. Unwin Seed Company, where she had been employed for seventy years. Mrs. Wilson had been among the firm's first women employees, and she had held her position until age 100. Her special relationship to the company dated back many decades to a time when, as a midwife, she had saved the life of the firm's present chairperson, grandson of its founder. She lived in Histon, some miles on the other side of Cambridgeshire, but she had attended Alice's 108th birthday party. The Tarrants spoke of still other lively centenarians and commented that most of them took an occasional drink. Without naming names, Norman Tarrant stated that at least one of the ladies over age 103 kept a bottle of brandy in her walking frame in case a nip was needed for a quick spurt of energy.

The phenomenon of having 3 centenarians under one roof and a cluster of even more centenarians in a small geographic area was a far cry from the time William Thoms had feared there might not be any genuine centenarians at all. The longevous ladies of Cambridgeshire also underscored the rapid rise in the number of British centenarians since the conclusion of World War II.

Additional information on what kind of people were becoming centenarians in a place like Cambridgeshire was available in local newspapers. From January, 1974, through September, 1978, the Cambridge *Evening News* published numerous stories, mainly obituaries and birthday coverage, concerning 37 centenarians. These included 33 local people, 2 visitors, and 2 individuals living elsewhere in Great Britain. Fourteen of the local centenarians could not be traced beyond a name and address, but backup material on the others was available through reporters, relatives, neighbors, medical personnel, and personal interviews.[9]

Thirty of the 33 local people were women—a percentage generally considered a consequence of the casualties suffered in the wars fought by Great Britain in the preceding hundred years. Of the 16 women for whom there were substantial data, 15 were from working-class or agricultural backgrounds. Most had worked as domestics at some time during their lives. The exception was Dame Harriet Chick, a professional nutritionist whose ideas about diet were similar to those of Sir Robert McCarrison. Most of the women and all of the men had been residents of the many rural hamlets characteristic of the region. Nine of the women had led lives that they or others considered vigorous. Sarah Fullard, for example, had taken many cycling trips around Great Britain with her father. More typical were the accounts of long walks to work. By 1978 the majority of the women were deceased, only a few of them having lived more than a short time past their 101st birthdays, but there were 4 still alive past age 104: Florence Jeaps, Rachel Rennie, Polly Wilson, and Alice Empelton.

The 3 male centenarians, Horace Williams, James Sellers, and Horace Bull, had slightly different collective profiles in terms of professions, having been, respectively, a headmaster, an accountant, and a butcher, but they had all been extremely vigorous individuals. Williams and Sellers had been cycling enthusiasts, the accountant often having stated that as a young Romeo he had frequently cycled from London to Cambridge to court the woman he eventually married. Horace Bull had devoted many of his later years to outdoor activities, presiding at sporting events and earning the title of Britain's eldest and most celebrated angler. At 99 he had climbed up on the roof of his cottage to make needed repairs, and he had celebrated his 100th birthday with a day of deep-sea fishing. Bull died at 101, of a virus which had made his housekeeper and daughter seriously ill as well. Before then, his housekeeper stated that Mr. Bull had given no indication of physical decline and was planning hunting and fishing trips in various parts of Great Britain.

The 2 centenarian visitors described by the press were Walter Terry, age 100, an active horse owner, and James Chapman, age 103, who had had tea with Mrs. Empelton. Since his retirement, Chapman had taken his first rides in an airplane, a glider, and a balloon. He was hoping to arrange for his first rides in a submarine and a helicopter. Two other centenarians written about were the deceased Sarah Ellen Morgan, age 111, the most recent British member of the exclusive superlongevous club, and lively Elizabeth Archer, age 100, who had made a stir with her annual trip to a Norfolk seaside holiday camp. Mrs. Archer had worked as a home helper until into her 80s and still did her own housework, mowed her own lawn, and gardened. She continued to enjoy a glass of sherry and liked to play bingo.

Both Sheringham and the Cambridgeshire hamlets provide instances in which the superior environment of past epochs persists amid the advantages of a highly developed modern nation. As elsewhere, the major ingredients for unusual life-spans appear to be a highly developed self-esteem, a lifelong history of physical activity, and a diet of common foods rich in natural nutrients. Sophisticated social services, skilled medical intervention, and rapid communications also have played a role in the British longevity boom. Most importantly, the high spirits of the British centenarians and the long life-spans recorded in Sheringham for more than two hundred years should be eye-openers for those who believe that lively long-living people can be found only in exotic locales.

7

RETHINKING THE FIRST NINETY-NINE

> For when they [the worthy young men] saw their parents and kindred snatcht away in the midst of their days and me contrarwise, at the age of eightie and one, strong and lustie; they had a great desire to know the way of my life . . .
>
> —*Luigi Cornaro*

Popular conceptions of what constitutes long life have had a dual character for at least two hundred years. The ultimate age one might aspire to has remained a little over 100 years, but the average life-span, greatly influenced by social factors, has been in constant flux, moving from the late 30s to the early 70s. As the twentieth century draws to an end, the double-tier pattern persists, but there is considerable misunderstanding about health expectations after 60. Because lifestyles vary so markedly, as the decades of life begin to mount the chronological age of individuals reveals less and less about their biological age. One septuagenarian will be able to row a lifeboat into a North Sea gale to help rescue a shipwrecked sailor, while a retiree of the same age can barely muster the energy to rise from a rocking chair. Most observers of the 2 septuagenarians would assume that the seaman has extended youth beyond the normal limits, yet it is really the retiree who is the biological anomaly.

The kind of vitality popularly associated with the age span of 40 to 60 can be extended to 80, with the decline thereafter even slower than that now generally seen in those over age 70. The only "secret" involved in this de facto extension by at least one-third of the most productive part of life is that unlike the case of a mechanical device which wears out more rapidly the more it is used, efficiency and power in living creatures decline when the organism is not constantly working. Any part of the human body that is neglected will begin to atrophy. Common instances of this are muscles which turn to fat and bones which become porous. Among sedentary populations, premature aging brought on by years of bodily neglect is one of the chief underlying causes of the majority of deaths.

How far even the healthiest octogenarians and non-agenarians are from enjoying the optimum potential of the human body is underscored by the medical cliché that there is no known case of a human being having perished strictly from old age. Such a diagnosis would require that all parts of the body had worn out more or less simultaneously, with death the result of general collapse and decrepitude. Instead of this scenario, death usually results from a specific disease, an injury, a systemic malfunction, or an organ failure. Given a cure for the disease, a healing of the injury, a repair of the malfunction, or a replacement of the organ, the body would have been capable of carrying on for many more years, if not decades.

The spectacular gain in the average life-span registered in the past two hundred years has barely touched on the extension of life beyond 85 or even on the curtailment of premature aging in the mature adult. Instead, the gains have come from a drastic lowering of the death rate among infants and children. To be more comprehensive: the records available from the Classic Age in Greece through to the early nineteenth century indicate that the average life-span in Europe has fluctuated between 20 and 40, the lower 30s being more common most of the time. Beginning around 1800, the average life-span began to rise. By the outset of the 1980s, it had reached the lower 70s for men and the higher 70s for women. During the same period, the predictable maximal life-span, the plateau at which almost all those born in the same year have perished, barely moved, remaining at about 80 to 85. This means that roughly one-half of the deaths of any given birth group occurred from the time of birth to the early 70s and the other half from that point to about age 85. Only a fraction lived on to become longevous. (The phenomenon of static maximal life expectancy can be concretized by a look at figures for the United States. From the time of the signing of the Declaration of Independence in 1776 to the census of 1970, the life expectancy for anyone able to reach 60 has remained constant, about fifteen to twenty years, with one lower point reached around 1900 and a higher one around 1945.)

Not a few commentators have recalled that three thousand years before the birth of Jesus, the Hebrew composer of the Ninetieth Psalm taught that the time on earth given to humans was three score and ten, with another decade for the hardy. This is an impressive historical precedent for believing there may be some kind of genetic ninth-decade barrier beyond which only a biological elite can penetrate. Among Soviet gerontologists it is a rule of thumb that only those persons in robust health at 85 are likely to become centenarians. Yet viewing the ninth decade as a barrier most humans cannot hope to surmount makes the error of treating the social forces that brought about the doubling of the average life-span as if they existed in sealed compartments.

In 1800 the leading causes of death were various infectious diseases. By the advent of the 1980s, none of them was among the major killers in the developed world. In their stead were the maladies poorly labeled as degenerative diseases, primarily cardiovascular diseases and the diseases collectively referred to as cancer. The three leading killers in the United States were diseases of the heart (38 percent), cancer (16 percent), and strokes (10.8 percent). When deaths from diabetes mellitus (2 percent), arteriosclerosis (1.7 percent), and cirrhosis of the liver (1.6 percent) are added in, the degenerative diseases accounted for more than 70 percent of all deaths. The percentages in the rest of the developed world were similar.[1]

The favored interpretation of these data is that during earlier historical periods infectious diseases killed off most of the population before it lived long enough to fall victim to the degenerative diseases. But this analysis has begun to collapse in the face of devastating cross-cultural evidence to the contrary. There are at least twenty-five entire nations, mostly in developing parts of the world, in which heart diseases and cancers remain rare at every age.

An explanation for the rise of degenerative diseases as killers in the developed world lies in what makes it developed: the triumph of the industrial revolution in the nineteenth century and the birth of its petrochemical and nuclear components in the twentieth. These far-reaching revolutions in the modes of production have brought about unprecedented alterations in the quality and nature of social relationships, of the work process, of the food chain, and of the general environment. The difference from preceding epochs is one of kind, not degree.

Owing to the thrilling successes against the menace of infectious diseases which took place concurrently with the production revolution, new man-made health threats have not been fully comprehended. But it is in the history of the struggle against infectious diseases that useful guidelines on how to war against degenerative diseases can be found. The magic bullets or vaccines developed by scientists, the cure approach, proved to be less crucial in the long run than vast public-health campaigns, the prevention approach. Once it was understood that microbes caused specific illnesses, societies moved to purify their water supplies, to improve their sewage-disposal systems, to upgrade public awareness of the importance of hygiene, and to isolate those suffering from communicable diseases. Fierce opposition to these measures came from entrenched forces, including doctors who could not admit past training was in error, industrialists resistant to lowering profit margins for reasons of health and safety, and politicians hesitant to budget allocations for public health. The most notorious example of obstinate resistance was the slow reform made in hospital procedures. Before the work of those brilliant investigators Paul de Kruif has called the microbe hunters, physicians blandly moved from one patient to another without washing their hands or sterilizing their instruments. Hospitals, which should have been citadels of healing, actually were major health hazards. The effect on the infant mortality rate was particularly tragic. Even after the carefully constructed demonstrations of Semmelweiss, it took decades to achieve the needed reforms.

The potential for dealing with infectious diseases was highlighted in 1978 when the World Health Organization was able to announce the eradication of smallpox. Except for laboratory samples, the germs that had once been the scourge of millions no longer existed on planet Earth. The victory was the consequence of an international campaign carried on for nearly two decades. Similar efforts aimed at other contagious diseases were in progress at various international, regional, and national levels. The eventual effect on average life-spans around the world could be spectacular. The newest magic bullets, like penicillin, antibiotics, and the polio vaccines, have not been in use long enough to have had a statistical impact on longevity figures in either the developed or the developing world. While it would be most premature to announce that the struggle against infectious diseases is over in any nation or area of the world, the tools for victory are in hand. Few well-informed persons in developed nations are in much danger of dying prematurely because of an infectious disease.

The prospects for avoiding degenerative diseases are less satisfying. The long rise in the incidence of heart diseases in the United States was not checked until the late 1970s, when the primary cause of most heart problems and their allied maladies finally was tied to diet and a slothful life-style. Heart specialists began to advocate dietary and exercise programs that were amazingly similar to those found in the biographies of longevous people. Consequently, heart disease, the foremost threat to individual longevity for most of the twentieth century, should decrease significantly among those willing to undertake the preventive regimens already established and constantly being improved upon.

Cancer prevention is more problematic and much less given to individual solution. If present assessments are correct, as much as 90 percent of all cancer, and certainly no less than 70 percent, is attributable to identifiable pollutants, mainly of petrochemical origin, in the air, water, food, and soil. The section in this book on the toxic society will deal with the problem in detail and outline steps an individual might take to minimize personal risk, but in the long run, only political action on at least the national level can make the environment as safe as it was during the time of Columbus. The menace posed by the toxic society is by far the most formidable and least controllable threat to individual longevity. It will be increasingly dangerous until such time as certain technological and chemical processes are totally rejected or rigidly supervised.

Just how many years would be added to the average life-span by the control of heart disease and cancer is conjectural, but the usual estimate is anywhere from twelve to twenty. This would bring the average life-span for both men and women to the doorstep of the tenth decade. Of course, there is no way of knowing if some presently unknown cluster of diseases might not emerge unexpectedly as still new barriers to long life, but there is no hint of such a development. The known degenerative diseases appear to be the last major obstacle in the path of a massive centenarian upsurge.

Quite as important as the damages inflicted by diseases are the declines brought about by normal wear and tear, and anyone interested in long life needs to understand that process in order to deal intelligently with the variables in the longevity agenda. In the United States, for example, by the age of 75, the average brain will weigh 8 percent less than at age 30, the nerve conduction velocity will be 10 percent slower, the cardiac output at rest 30 percent less, the kidney filtration rate 31 percent slower, and the breathing capacity 57 percent less.[2] Such dramatic declines would appear to indicate a substantially weakened organism, yet, because of genetic overprogramming, this is not exactly the case. The kidneys provide an excellent demonstration. It is possible for an individual to live in good health on one kidney operating at 50-percent efficiency. Given that even at age 75 the average decline of 31 percent is spread over two kidneys, there remains a wide margin of safety. This kind of reserve capacity is found in all systems, and a conditioned body will experience significantly less decline than that recorded in composite averages.

A decline that is difficult to combat and will cause long-term health woes for those unwilling to deal with it is the slowing basal metabolic rate. After 30, if a person continues to consume the same number of calories while maintaining the same level of physical activity as previously, there will be a gradual weight gain, almost all of which will be fat. This new weight increases demands on the body's maintenance systems at the very time they are becoming less efficient. This may explain to some degree the positive correlation found between excess weight and susceptibility to virtually all diseases. The countermeasure to this process is to consume fewer calories as one grows older and/or to become physically more active, the opposite of what generally happens in a society such as the United States, particularly after a person "retires."

Problems brought on by overweight are hardly confined to the old. From 1900 onward, the national average weight in the United States has steadily increased. Even in the 1970s, when many Americans began to shed excess pounds as part of a renewed enthusiasm for physical fitness, the national average weight increased by more than 6 pounds. It seems that the portion of the population which was getting heavier was doing so at a faster rate than the portion that was becoming lighter. If that is so, premature death influenced by excess weight might hold down future rises in the average life-span while the maximal life expectancy begins to move upward—a shift in the pattern of the past two centuries. That this may be happening already is indicated by the observation that the population arriving at 70 seems to be in better physical shape than previous groups at that plateau and by the general belief that there is an increase in the total octogenarian population which is not accounted for by the slowly rising average life-span. The 1980 census analysis will provide important insights into this development.

Whatever one's weight or age, the quality of health ultimately depends upon a vibrant cellular life, which in turn is related to the availability of oxygen to burn food and release energy. Since oxygen cannot be stored in the body, fresh supplies must be breathed in constantly and shipped via the bloodstream to waiting cells. Unless the capacities of the two major bodily pumps, the lungs and the heart, are maintained through vigorous and appropriate aerobic activities, the availability of oxygen will decline substantially. This will accelerate the deterioration in vital organs, as they must work harder to perform their normal functions. Thus, the importance of respiratory and cardiovascular health would be difficult to exaggerate. They affect the proper functioning of the body from relatively minor tasks like keeping the toes warm to the essential job of maintaining the power of the brain.

Senility, one of the greatest fears of old age, is thought to be caused at least in part by oxygen deficiency in the brain brought on by arterial blockages of the same types that produce heart attacks. Yet even with the mediocre cardiovascular health of the general population, only 1 percent will ever be diagnosed as senile, a percentage that is less than the number of people who will go insane at earlier ages. In addition, many persons believed to be senile actually suffer from reversible psychological depression or vitamin deficiencies.[3]

Fear of senility touches on the assumption that mental ability dulls with age. The available evidence offers little proof for such a contention. Achievement tests administered to older people show little change from scores made on earlier tests, and in the case of scholars there is frequently a gain. Follow-up discussions about test taking have indicated that as a group, older people are not very enthusiastic about challenges which have no practical purpose or promise of individual benefit. Often they have had unpleasant experiences with bureaucrats in which volunteered information has been used against their interests. A subsequent lack of eagerness to cooperate with strangers, who are usually affiliated with the government, or with educational bodies may reflect a shrewd defense posture as much as any expression of stubbornness or fear of failure.

A potent indicator that mental abilities need not decline with age is the number of individuals over 70 who have made extraordinary contributions to human culture. The percentages may very well be *higher* than those at most other age levels. Authors of advanced years have written many of the works that would appear on any list of the hundred best books ever written by Europeans. Cervantes completed *Don Quixote* at age 69, Goethe finished *Faust* at 83, and Sophocles was in his late 80s when he wrote the final plays in the Oedipus cycle. Two of the best surveys of men and women who did outstanding work after age 70 are those done by Harvey Lehman and Ruth Hubbell.[4] They have surprisingly few duplications, yet with their focus on the fine arts and theoretical science, many exceptional individuals are excluded. Neither list, for example, was designed to include a political figure like Mother Jones, who was socially active throughout her 90s, wrote a spirited autobiography at age 95, and attended her last May Day rally on her 100th birthday, some months before her death.

The life of Mother Jones also shows how fallacious it is

to assume that humans become politically more conservative and generally more cautious as they grow older. Studies of the longevous show that just the opposite is often true. Many of the social pressures felt at other ages seem less important or are thought to be irrelevant. In Abkhasia, we saw how women of advanced years grew bolder and more liberated the older they got. The old are often so direct and uncompromising in their views that they are accused of being gruff, garrulous, or crude. On a more sophisticated level, persons with strong social commitments usually pursue their visions to the end of their lives, often spurred on by the notion that the time left to make changes is short. Two remarkable examples are Bertrand Russell and Welthy Honsinger Fisher.

World-famous as a philosopher and long forgiven his pacifism, in 1960, at the age of 88, Bertrand Russell formed the Committee of One Hundred to fight the threat of nuclear annihilation. His ban-the-bomb group was a breakaway from a more conservative organization, and its tactics of civil disobedience were to be adopted throughout the developed world by various political movements of the 1960s. In the last ten years of his life, Russell interceded in the Cuban missile crisis with appeals to the heads of the Soviet and American governments, and he launched a tribunal to investigate the charges of American war crimes in Vietnam. During the same time span he completed a three-volume autobiography, whose sales helped finance his many interests.

The name of Welthy Fisher does not have the same recognition factor, yet she typifies many people dedicated to religious or humanitarian causes. Having given up a promising career in opera to become a missionary, she spent eleven years in China teaching at a school that became a prototype for women's education. After her return to the West in 1917, Fisher continued to work on various programs of the Methodist Church, always being noted for her feminist and antiracist point of view. She married at age 44, but although her husband was a highly placed church official, she did not curb her independent commitments. In 1947 she met Mahatma Gandhi, an old friend of her deceased husband's, and she was persuaded to begin a school in India much like the one she had run in China. Following years of preparation, in 1956, at the age of 77, Welthy opened Literacy House on a 23-acre site in Lucknow. Twenty-two years later, suffering from a broken kneecap and facing sub-zero temperatures, she accepted an invitation for a return visit to China. Now 99 years of age, she consulted with Madame Sun Yat-sen and others she had known from her missionary days about the progress Chinese women had been making toward a goal of full social equality. Interviewed on her return, Fisher made a statement that could be the credo of many longevous people who share her spirit even though their lives might be less spectacular: "I could never manage to feel as I was supposed to about my chronological age. Maybe I was too busy. The future always seemed limitless and I have never stopped expecting something to happen, some invitation for another adventure."[5] On September 18, 1979, at a birthday dinner for 250 friends, at the St. Regis Hotel in New York, Welthy Honsinger Fisher became a centenarian.

Complementing accounts of those who reach the summit of their careers in old age are others about those who embark on new careers or new phases of old ones. Artists and scholars provide many examples. Thomas Hardy, already enshrined as one of the greatest English novelists, began to concentrate on writing outstanding poetry from his mid-60s onward. In like manner, after reaching their 70s, Claude Monet began his famous lily-pond series, and Henrik Ibsen changed his literary style. Writers from Cato to Somerset Maugham have insisted that the 80s are a splendid time to start the study of a new language. Other individuals have embarked on entirely new forms of personal expression late in life. When already well into her 70s, Anna Mary Moses found that her fingers were becoming too stiff to hold a needle to embroider on canvas as had been her custom. Although the former farm woman was unschooled, she decided to concentrate on her oil painting. Before long, she had become world-famous as Grandma Moses, "the grand old lady of American art." She continued to be an active artist until several months before her death at age 101. Among her final works were illustrations done at age 100 for a new edition of *A Visit from St. Nicholas.*

About the only area of mental competence in which there appears to be a significant incidence of degeneration is near memory. This condition can be redressed through mental exercises if an individual is concerned, and experiments with choline indicate that some vitamins can foster better near and remote memory, even though most older people have little difficulty with the latter.[6] Older persons who keep their minds engaged in activities such as crossword puzzles, complex card games, chess, and personal finances have been observed to suffer far less from loss of memory than those who are intellectually more passive.[7] Moreover, memory and rote-learning abilities decline much less in persons with a formal education—indicating, perhaps, that many tests measure test-taking "savvy" as much as raw mental capacity.

The circumstances surrounding loss of memory can be extremely critical. When a busy executive forgets something, it is chalked up to overwork. The same memory lapse in the old may be considered a sign of approaching senility. It is common for people to forget to buy an item on their shopping list, to misplace keys, or to hide an important document so cleverly that they forget where it is themselves. If an older person becomes depressed or withdrawn by fears that such typical human behavior is a signal of mental decline, the fear may become self-fulfilling.

The advantages of keeping the mind constantly stimulated can be seen by the large numbers of people who remain active in the business or political worlds long after the typical retirement age. Senior partners in law firms, brokerage houses, and business enterprises who are in their 80s or beyond are legendary. Adolph Zukor, founder of Paramount

Pictures, continued to visit the studio to give advice on projects until his death at 103. Still more common has been the number of older men found in the judicial and executive branches of government. In the United States, 85 percent of Supreme Court service has been rendered by men over 65. It is well known that Oliver Wendell Holmes was a justice until age 91, but this is still fifteen years shy of the world record held by Judge Albert R. Alexander, who remained on the Missouri bench until nearly 106. In the matter of chief executives, every nation in the developed world has had at least one head of state since 1940 who was 70 years of age or older. The *Guinness Book of World Records* asserts the oldest recorded head of state to be El Hadji Mohammed of Mokri, Grand Vizier of Morocco, who died in 1957 at the reputed age of 112. The oldest member of a parliament is Jozsef Madarasz (1814–1915) of Hungary, who was in office at the time of his death.

Anxieties over failing hearing are more justified than fear of mental lethargy. Fully 27 percent of those over 65 will suffer some such impairment; but again, the most serious aspect of the problem is psychological. People who have hearing difficulty may withdraw into a private world because they are scorned or ridiculed when they fail to reply to unheard questions or give lucid but inappropriate responses to misheard questions. Clearly, a person living with loved ones stands a better chance of avoiding this kind of depression than someone in an overcrowded institution, and advances in hearing technology have provided less cumbersome and more sensitive aids than the old hearing horns which tended to make the user appear somewhat ridiculous.

It is also necessary to emphasize that the majority of persons over 65 will not have serious hearing loss and will continue to enjoy their fill of conversation and music. Older musicians have as impressive a list of new works as older writers do. Verdi, for one, composed *Otello* at 73, *Falstaff* at 80, and completed his *Quattro Pezzi Sacri (Four Sacred Pieces)* at 85. Wagner completed *Parsifal* at age 69, and

Richard Strauss wrote his poignant *Four Last Songs* at age 85. In the period since the end of World War II there have been numerous octogenarian and nonagenarian musicians who continued to perform on the concert stage. Three of the most notable nonagenarians were conductor Leopold Stokowski, pianist Artur Rubinstein, and cellist Pablo Casals.

Decline in the ability to see, signaled by the need for reading glasses, a norm in developed nations, is not a prelude to blindness. Few of the old become blind, and most of these cases are caused by cataracts, which could have been operated on if diagnosed early. Like so many physical declines, problems with eyesight appear to be due less to simple aging than to environment, which in this instance means reading and working under artificial illumination. Dramatic support of how important this factor may be is available in studies of Eskimo culture, in which it was found that individuals who lived in the traditional manner experienced little eyesight decline, while those who installed light bulbs in their dwellings developed high rates of myopia in less than a generation.

Professional artists, like hundreds of thousands of amateurs, usually find that failing eyesight is not a barrier to their creativity. Pablo Picasso was doing an ongoing series of erotic works in his 80s, and during the Renaissance Titian was busy on mythological paintings until his death at 99. Active nonagenarian graphic artists on the contemporary scene would include Marc Chagall and Georgia O'Keeffe. Among the most notable achievements by visual artists of advanced age was the work done by Michelangelo Buonarroti, who was carving the Rondanini *Pietà* almost to the day of his death at age 89. During the last two decades of his life, he had worked as a painter and architect as well, designing the Piazza del Campidoglio, painting the frescoes in the Cappella Paolina, and designing the apse and dome of the Basilica of Saint Peter.

Many misconceptions regarding the old stem from the common practice of saying a person does or does not look his or her age. As there is no way that visual observation, even by an expert, can determine the ages of people from 60 to 100 years old, this kind of statement is meaningless. It simply associates ill health and a poor appearance with advanced chronological age. More errors accumulate when impressions are based on the performance of the 5 percent of the population over 65 who are institutionalized rather than on the 95 percent who are not.[8] Many are in institutions because of ill health, poverty, or abandonment. Their responses to survey questions and their scores on achievement tests might be considerably different if they were living at home in relative health. In view of this, all statistical data derived from institutionalized populations must be considered as presenting minimal rather than aggregate portraits of the abilities of the old and longevous.

A look at longevity that excluded persons in institutions was offered by Dr. Stephen Jewett in 1973.[9] Over the years, using informal means of contact, Jewett had managed to locate and keep track of 70 persons between the ages of 85 and 103. The majority of his 70 subjects had remained active throughout their lives and were independently employed, mainly being farmers, professionals, or owners of small enterprises. They were moderate eaters, their diets being light in fat and heavy in protein. They were not overweight, used little medication, and reported few colds. As a rule, the few who drank and smoked did so moderately. There was a high rate of marriage, and there was excellent sociability. Most reported they were not prone to worry and slept well. Their nonstressful style of life included taking periodic but brief vacations and occasionally experimenting with new foods.

Findings similar to those described by Jewett appear in a survey completed in the 1960s of 402 Americans over age 95.[10] These nonagenarians had moderate habits, had worked at jobs they liked, had not been big eaters, had enjoyed plenty of physical exercise, and had retained their zest for living through activities ranging from hobbies and money management to participating in extended families. While both this

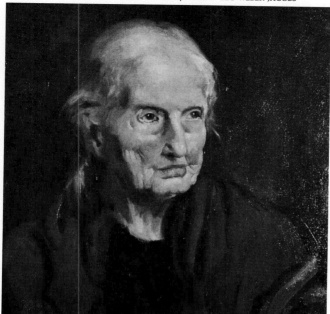

Delina Filkins (1815–1928) of Herkimer, New York, is the longest-lived documented female.

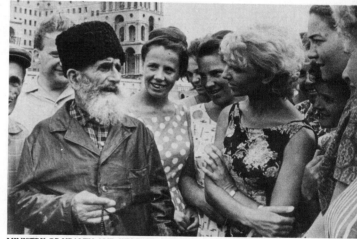

Shirali Mislimov of Barzavu, Azerbaijan, died in 1973 at the reputed age of approximately 170.

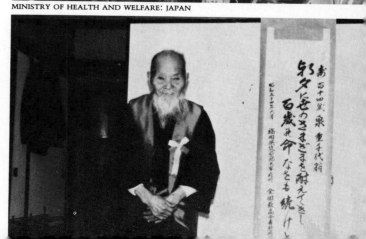

Shigechiyo Izumi (June 29, 1865–) of Japan is accepted as the longest-living human being by the *Guinness Book of World Records.*

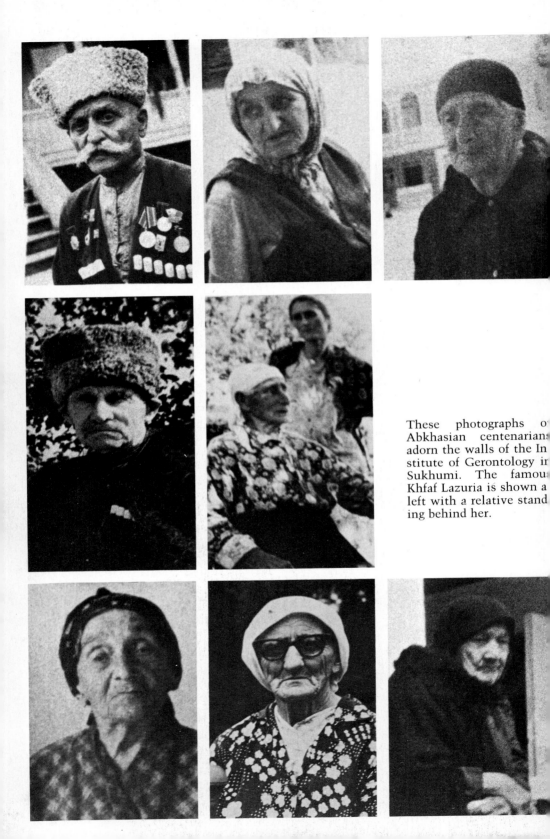

These photographs of Abkhasian centenarians adorn the walls of the Institute of Gerontology in Sukhumi. The famous Khfaf Lazuria is shown at left with a relative standing behind her.

The author toasts Van-
acha Temur, age 110.
Temur is identified by
Abkhasian authoritie as
one of their healthiest
centenarians. His two-
story house is built in the
style typical of the region.
The topography of Ab-
khasia becomes hilly to
mountainous a few miles
inland from the Black
Sea.

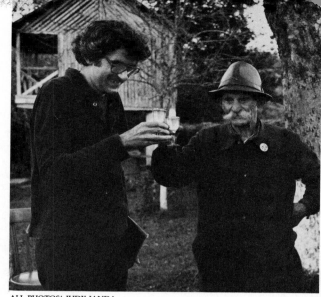

ALL PHOTOS: JUDY JANDA

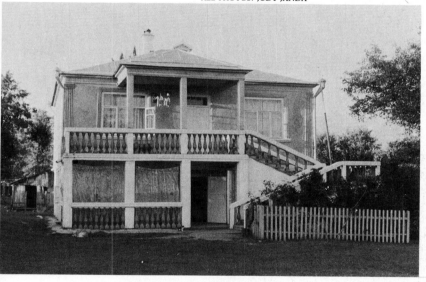

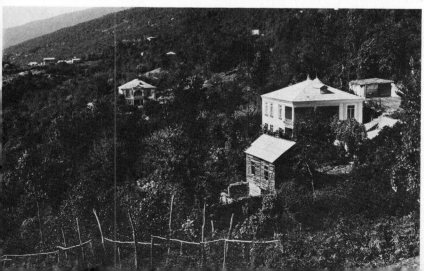

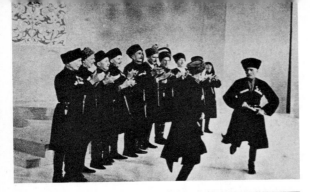

A person must be at least 70 years old to be eligible for membership in this choir.

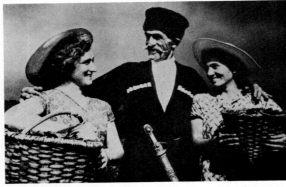

Opposite, Mikhail Kaslantzia, age 103, and his wife looking at photographs of centenarians in other parts of the world.

This Soviet photograph is used in a poster to encourage people to work as hard as their elders did.

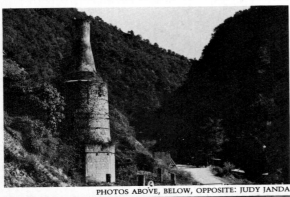

Towers of the Great Abkhasian Wall (11th century) can be found in the rugged Abkhasian countryside.

Dr. Shoto Gogoghian, Director of the Institute of Gerontology in Sukhumi, explains longevity charts to author · and interpreter.

PHOTOS ABOVE, BELOW, OPPOSITE: JUDY JANDA

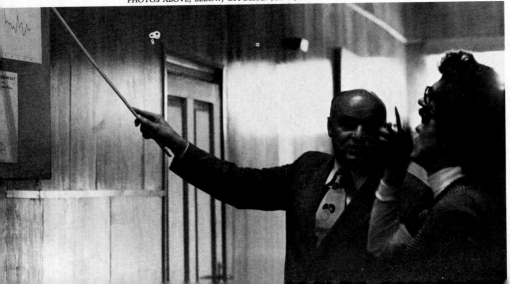

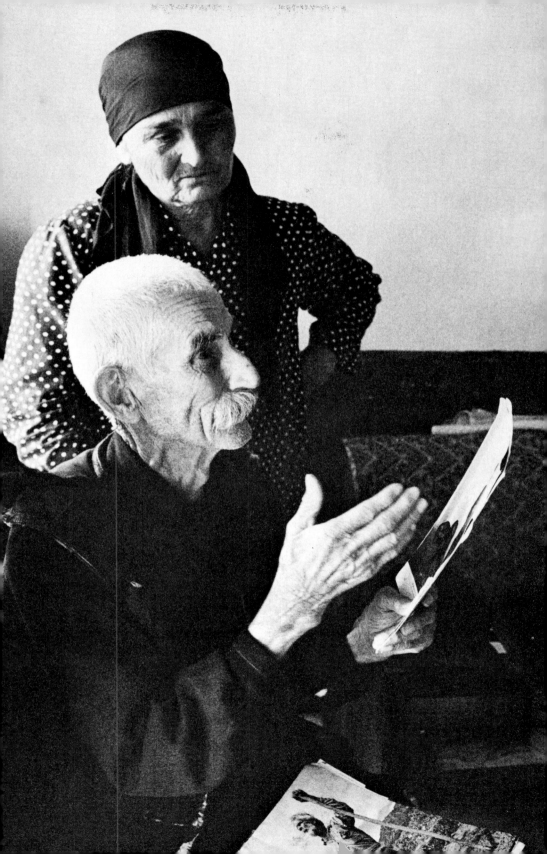

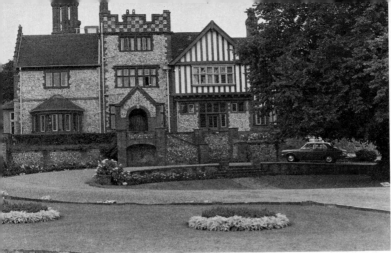

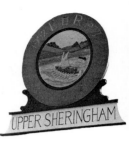

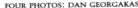

FOUR PHOTOS: DAN GEORGAKAS

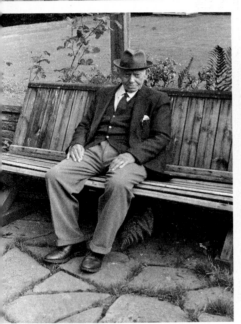

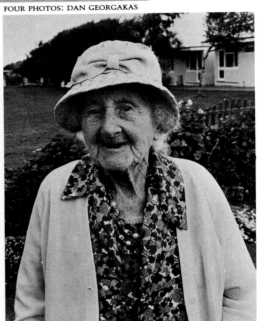

EASTERN DAILY PRESS

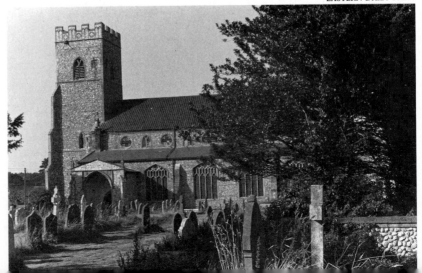

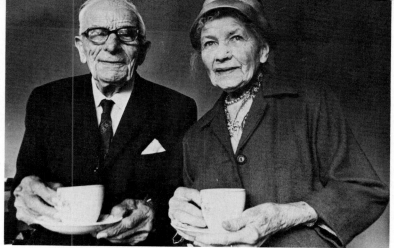

OPPOSITE PAGE:

Top, The Dales belongs to a category of homes in Britain operated for seniors who can manage most of their daily tasks unaided. *Center left*, at age 104, Frederick Cornelius of Upper Sheringham traveled alone by bus and taxi. *Center right*, Elizabeth Archer celebrated her 100th birthday at a seaside holiday camp in Norfolk. *Bottom*, long lives recorded on these tombstones led to a belief that there was unusual longevity in Upper Sheringham, Great Britain.

THIS PAGE:

Top, while traveling in the Cambridge area, James Chapman, age 103, had tea with Alice Empelton, also 103 at the time of the photograph. *Right*, Alice Empelton continued to garden until she was nearly 106. *Below*, Rachel Rennie, age 104, chats with Alice shortly after Mrs. Empelton's 108th birthday.

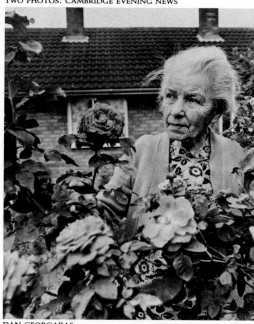

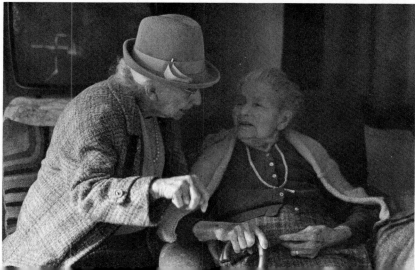

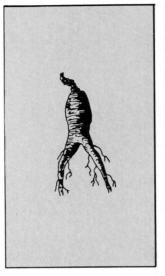

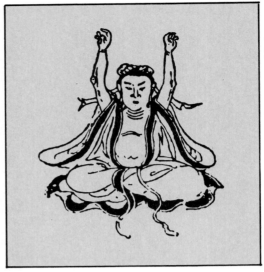

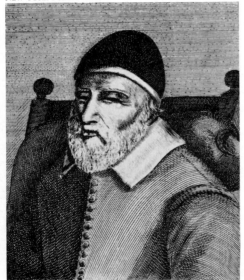

Above left, ginseng is among the rare plants mistakenly thought to increase the life span.

Above right, elaborate regimens like the Taoist longevity exercise shown here are less likely to aid longevity than vigorous daily walking.

Left, Thomas Parr's claim of 152 years of life (1483–1635), accepted for more than a century, has long been shown to be false.

Below, Charles Smith became a celebrity during the last twenty years of his life because of his claim to an extraordinarily long life of more than 115 years.

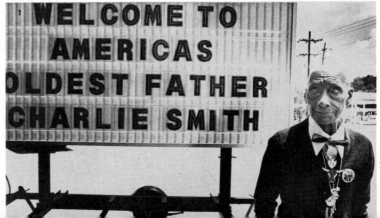

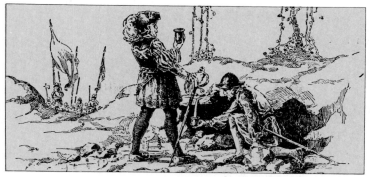

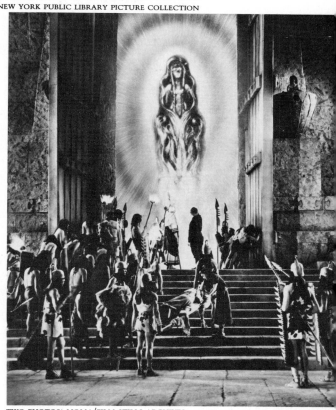

Longevous utopias have always been thought to exist at the edge of the known world. *Above,* Ponce de Leon thought a Fountain of Youth flowed in the then New World of North America. *Right,* H. Rider Haggard's *She* places a longevous meteor pit in a desolate region of Africa. *Below,* James Hilton's Himalayan Shangri-La, later confused with the kingdom of Hunza, could be reached only by a treacherous ice-laden path.

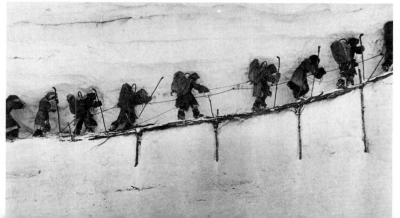

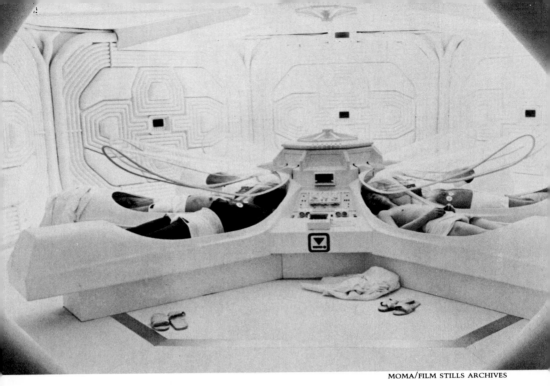

Science fiction ideas such as the suspended-animation tanks in *The Alien*, shown above, are beginning to emerge as science fact. For example, the cryonics movement hopes to freeze people shortly after death for revival at some future date. Shown below is a body about to be frozen in liquid nitrogen.

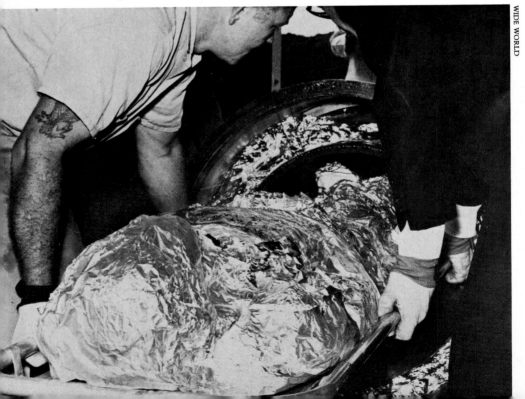

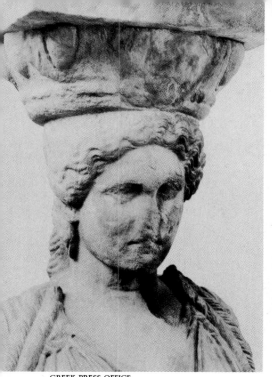

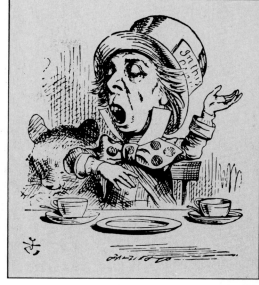

GREEK PRESS OFFICE

Environmental hazards to long life are symbolized by the smog-shrouded Gateway Arch in St. Louis (*below*) and the damage done to the Athenian Acropolis (*above*) by acidic rain. Lewis Carroll's Mad Hatter is based on the threat to mental health posed in the workplace by the mercury that hat makers use in the tanning process.

UPI

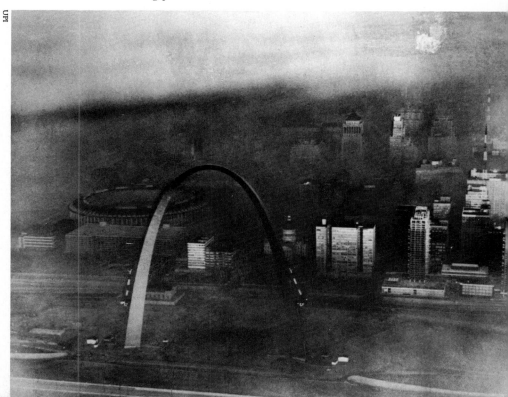

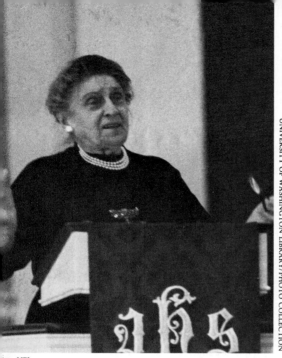

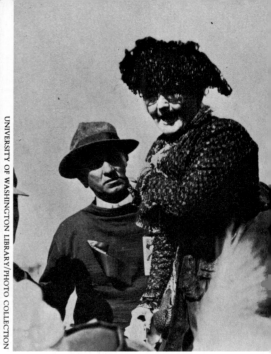

Above left, Welthy Fisher, shown here at age 90, traveled to China at age 99 and at age 100 was helping her secretary update her biography. *Above right*, Mother Jones argued for her causes throughout her long life, marching in her last May Day parade at the age of 100. *Below left*, Judge Albert R. Alexander, shown here filing for reelection at age 102, served until nearly 106. *Below right*, Basco Belasques, age 92, and two co-workers set a world's record by sorting 8,200 metal bars in an 8-hour shift at the Bethlehem Steel plant in 1973.

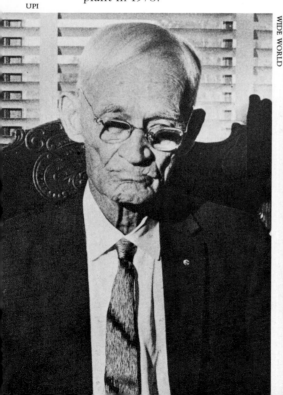

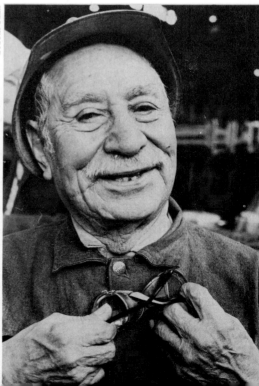

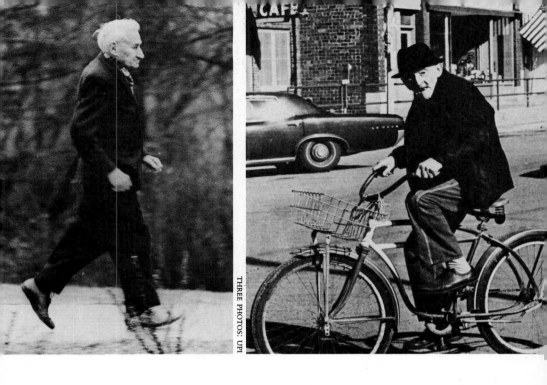

Above left, Leonard Shore, age 96, showing good jogging form. *Above right*, Martin Mack, age 105, uses his bicycle to deliver groceries. *Below left*, Fred Broadwell, age 95, taking a turn at bat. *Below right*, Maude Andrews, age 100, performing an exercise routine she has followed for decades.

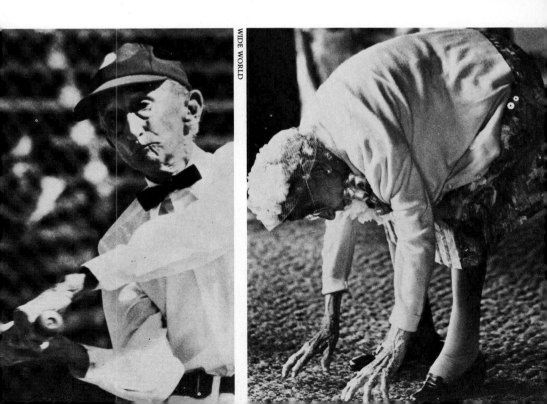

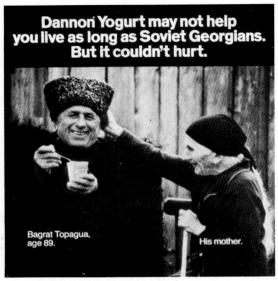

Dannon Yogurt may not help
you live as long as Soviet Georgians.
But it couldn't hurt.

Bagrat Topagua,
age 89.

His mother.

Above, an advertising campaign by the Dannon Yogurt Company capitalized on the belief that sour milk products are the secret of long life in Soviet Georgia. *Below left*, Luigi Cornaro (1467–1565) thrived on and wrote about his restricted diet of about a thousand calories a day. *Below right*, in 1959, Barbara Moore, age 56, walked from San Francisco to New York City in 85 days to demonstrate the energy and strength that she derived from her strict vegetarian diet.

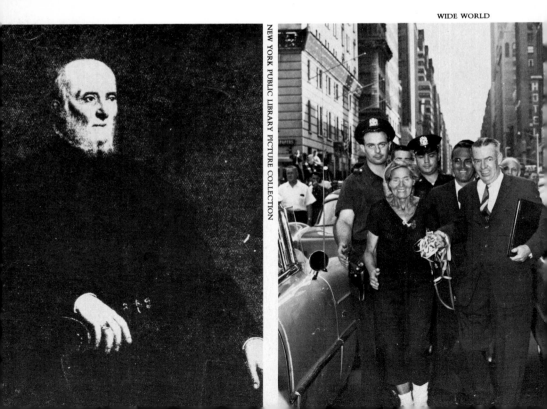

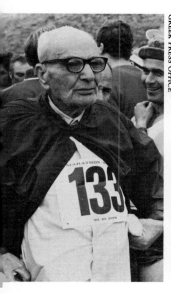

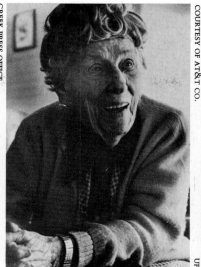

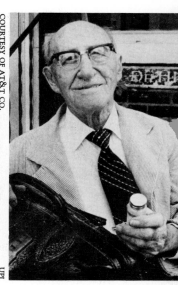

Above left, Demetrios Iordanidis, age 98, shown here before running in a 26.2 mile marathon, which he completed. *Above center*, in 1978, Dolly Warren, age 106, was hailed as the oldest of the three million owners of American Telephone & Telegraph stock. *Above right*, Talbert Hill celebrated his 100th birthday by calling an end to a 76-year medical practice. *Below left*, Lulu Sadler Craig, age 102, spoke eloquently of the Old West in a television documentary, "Happy Birthday, Mrs. Craig!" *Below right*, Grandma Moses produced works until a few months before her death at age 101.

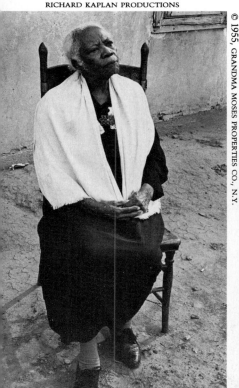

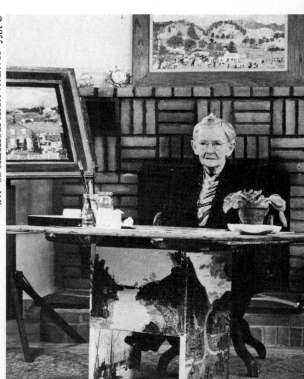

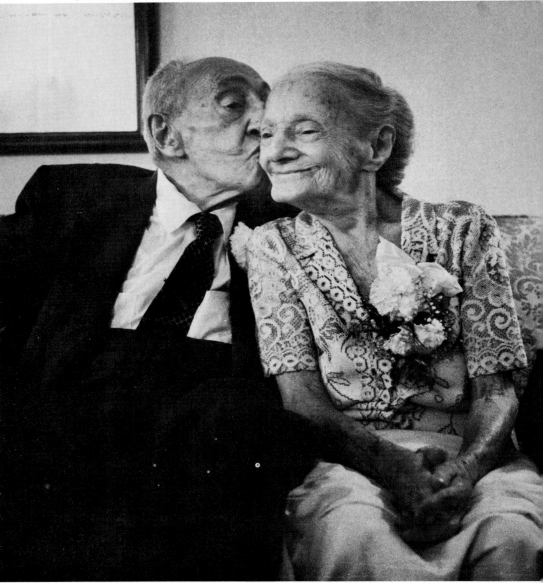

Julius Kahn, age 99, kissing his wife, Della, as they celebrated her 100th birthday on August 16, 1978, in New York City.

survey and Jewett's were too small and random to be more than supportive of other more methodical and comprehensive work, such as that done in the Soviet Union, the profile they describe corresponds more closely to the realizable biological possibilities for humans than do stereotypes of old-timers vegetating on the nursing-home veranda. All this work is also in line with physical-fitness programs in which men in their 70s and 80s were brought up to the performance levels of men in their 40s and 50s.[11]

The activist longevity profile is repeated in the writings of authors on longevity who, following their own precepts, lived to at least a tenth decade and wrote about it. Five of the most celebrated of this group are Luigi Cornaro, Sir Hermann Weber, Sir James Crichton-Browne, Dr. Alexandre Guéniot, and Scott Nearing. Cornaro and Nearing sought to share their philosophical vision of how life could be better for all the species, while Weber, Crichton-Browne, and Guéniot were physicians interested in promoting general health concepts.

By far the most celebrated of the quintet is Luigi Cornaro, who is generally believed to have been born in Venice in 1467 and to have died in Padua in 1565. Some authorities think he may have been born a few years earlier and did not die until 1566, making him a centenarian. Accepting the birth date of 1467, it can be said that Cornaro wrote his major treatise on longevity at age 83 and then revised the work at ages 86, 91, and 95. The discourse has been translated into every major European language. One early American rendition which appeared at the beginning of the nineteenth century carried an endorsement by George Washington.[12]

Until the age of 40, Cornaro had suffered from various maladies, such as gout, stomach fever, cold temperatures, and generalized pain. His physicians held out little hope for his survival. At this juncture, Cornaro decided to become his own healer, embarking upon a regimen that was to carry him through more than another fifty years of life. He had become convinced that his ills, like those of the human race in general, were due to a life of intemperance, to homage to "the belly gods" and the "nervous" life they commanded. He reformed his living habits, gradually cutting back on his eating until it came to only 12 ounces of solids, mainly eggs and flour products, and 14 ounces of young wine—a total of about 1,000 calories—a day. His body grew extremely lean, yet his health began to prosper.

Aside from his dietary experiments, Cornaro's life was typical of the upper-class male of the Italian Renaissance. He had a country estate, to which he frequently rode on horseback. More than casually interested in his property, Cornaro had swamplands drained and personally supervised the management of his crops. When in Padua, he participated in the intellectual currents of the day and spoke about the joy of long life. His many works include a comedy written in his 80s as a conscious challenge to the opinion that old age is dreary. His granddaughter, a nun, wrote that to the end of his life, when a meal might consist of a single egg yolk, Cornaro still liked to sing and possessed a strong, clear voice.[13]

The apparent dichotomy between the vigor of Cornaro's life and the meagerness of his diet has fascinated researchers for centuries. Perhaps as he grew older he exaggerated how little he ate or honestly forgot the fruits consumed in summer or the vegetables sliced into his soup. The tale of the egg-yolk dinner, like the effort to make him a centenarian, has the ring of apocrypha. Nevertheless, Cornaro's handling of a slowing basal metabolic rate and his whole approach to eating were in accord with the biological maxim developed in the twentieth century that the closer an organism comes to its minimal daily requirements, the longer it will endure. The classic experiment leading to this conclusion was made in the 1920s by Dr. Clive McCay of Cornell, who discovered that he could extend the life-span of laboratory rats from the usual 965 days to a little over 1,450 days by reducing their caloric intake to just above the starvation level.[14] For maximal benefit, it was necessary for the restricted diet to commence at birth and to contain all the nutrients required to maintain systemic efficiency. Subsequent experiments on other animals in laboratories all over the world have repeatedly brought the same general results.

Moral considerations prohibit massive tests on human subjects, but history has provided some gratuitous episodes that reproduce some aspects of the experiments linking dietary restriction to longevity. During both the world wars when food supplies, particularly of those high in fat content, were curtailed severely in various European countries, the death rates fell.[15] As soon as the normal diet was restored at the conclusion of hostilities, the death rates rebounded to their prewar levels. Prisoners in various camps where the food was minimal but not at starvation levels experienced no physical ill effects, and many reported cures of gastrointestinal ailments. For decades, one of the boasts of the officials of Moscow's Lubianka Prison was that the black-bread-and-fish diet served to their prisoners promoted good health.

The danger in a dietary approach such as Cornaro's is that if carried to an extreme, it can lead to starvation. This is the sad fate of persons afflicted with anorexia nervosa. Otherwise, however, it is not very likely in developed nations, where overeating seeds so many health problems. Unfortunately, in nearly every culture both the folk tradition and the fine arts associate fatness with the positive human qualities. Shakespeare's Caesar trusted only the well fed, and crazed Don Quixote was thin as a reed while his jovial comrade Sancho Panza was as plump as the bon vivants of Rabelais and the genial toy makers of fairy tales. Certainly during eras when famine was a real threat, fat served the useful function of providing a reservoir of emergency fuel, and historically, bulging bellies have been signs of prosperity. It also is readily seen that people who are seriously ill will suffer drastic weight loss. Nonetheless, the folk and literary sages are wrong to link overweight to a happy and long life. As noted before, there is a positive correlation between excess weight and susceptibility to nearly every disease; and the greater the excess, the greater the risk. It has been suggested that the longevity superiority of women is due to nothing more than that they are generally smaller and lighter than men. Whether this is a valid thesis or not, the lean and hungry look of Luigi Cornaro is standard in the longevity profile, particularly for those who live beyond the 95th year.

The role of wine, long called the milk of the old, in Cornaro's diet is another historical fluke that has proved to have a scientific basis. Massive statistical evidence gathered in the twentieth century shows that people who drink about half a liter of wine a day live longer than those who do not drink at all or those who drink wine in much larger quantities or those who drink alcohol in other forms.[16] It may be of significance that Cornaro liked young, local wine, for sulfur dioxide, which is added to make wines travel better, is suspected of being harmful to the body. There would be no reason to add it to local wines meant to be consumed quickly.

The independent yet reasonable spirit of Cornaro is another characteristic found frequently in the longevous. Unlike those who adhered blithely to the fashions of the age, Cornaro had the strength of character to persist in his own regimen, but with a temperament that did not alienate him from contemporaries. Like most of the longevous, Cornaro never "retired." At most there was a gradual easing in the tempo of his life after age 80, with less time spent on the estate and more on writing. Although his peers thought him extremely unusual, what moderns would call a "character," his good humor, his responsible behavior, and then his age made him one of the pillars of Paduan society. Like the advice of an Abkhasian elder, his counsel was sought and given on every subject.

Some four hundred years after the time of Cornaro, 3 European physicians of immense contemporary fame made longevity one of their major concerns. The longevity profiles they advocated were similar to that of Cornaro, but with a shift in major emphasis away from diet to physical activity. Each of the 3 doctors had seen numerous longevous patients as part of his practice, and they all capped their professional writing with books or essays on longevity composed or revised when they themselves were in their 90s.[17]

Sir Hermann Weber (1823–1918) was the most adamant about the role of exercise and was among the first to stress the added advantage of difficult terrain. He recommended from one to three hours of walking each day and taking vacations that included climbing, hiking, and hunting. Sir James Crichton-Browne (1840–1938) cited with favor that Cardinal de Satis, who lived to be 110, insisted on a mixture of two hours of walking and riding daily. Crichton-Browne underscored the advantages of vigorous country living and continuing projects throughout the life cycle. Across the Channel in Paris, Alexandre Guéniot (1832–1935) added a light Gallic touch to similar views by disclosing that before working on his present book at age 99 he had, as usual, reached his apartment by walking up fifty-six steps.

In regard to diet, Crichton-Browne believed that Cornaro's caloric intake was inadequate for the average person, although he conceded that it must always be related to the caloric output demanded by an individual's occupation and life-style. Expressing similar sentiments, Weber estimated that 2,500 calories was sufficient for the vast majority of people—a level about a thousand lower than Crichton-Browne's recommendations. As opposed to longevity per se, Weber argued that his regimen promoted a life-span in which death, whenever it came, would not be preceded by a prolonged period of suffering. Massages and deep-breathing exercises were highly thought of by Weber and Guéniot, respectively, as means of stimulating vital systems, and both favored a lactovegetarian diet. All 3 physicians were advocates of moderation in all things and were contemptuous of those who allowed themselves to fall ill at such tender ages as 60 and 70. Serving food at room temperature, keeping active throughout life, attention to personal hygiene, consumption of wine, and fostering an easygoing personality were other shared recommendations.

The contemporary American heir to the longevity mantle is Scott Nearing (1883–   ), who, like Cornaro, has become a legend in his own lifetime. The impetus to what Nearing labels living the good life involves a world outlook that encompasses controversial views on many basic social issues. Alone or in coauthorship with his wife, Helen (1904–   ), Nearing has written prolifically about his pacifist, vegetarian, and socialist beliefs. As a young man, Nearing had been an activist in the socialist movement, but by the end of the 1920s he began to think that the best way to reshape the world might be to forge a life-style which already contained as many of the values he advocated as possible. In 1932, he and Helen purchased a farm in Vermont, where they embarked on a living scheme that presaged many of the alternative-culture values which became popular some forty years later.

The Nearings' views on longevity are scattered throughout their writings but form an integral part of both *Living the Good Life,* an account of their nineteen years of homesteading in Vermont, and *Continuing the Good Life,* a report on the succeeding twenty-five years of homesteading in Maine.[18] The core of the Nearing life-style is to plan daily and seasonal chores in a manner that maximizes the amount of time available for activities not required for survival— what the Nearings call bread labor. Built into this approach are concerns for exercise, diet, and social involvement.

Having farmed mainly with hand implements for the better part of fifty years, the Nearings think formal exercise is a kind of folly as there is always productive work that can accomplish the same health goal. Major work done on their homestead includes digging, hoeing, weeding, composting, and hauling. In addition, Scott likes to saw and chop wood for their wood-burning stove, an activity he finds more enjoyable than any sport. An indication of the lust for activity that is part of the Nearing perspective is that one of their favorite leisure-time activities is building stone structures under a schema devised by Ernest Flagg. They have constructed fifteen stone buildings on their two homesteads, including two impressive stone houses. In typical Nearing fashion, they design the structure, quarry the stone, dig up the materials needed for cement, and erect the buildings with minimal outside assistance or machinery. Scott calls them one-man/one-woman projects, and Helen admits that she became so involved in the Maine house that she personally selected and placed every stone. That home was completed in 1977, when Scott was 94 and Helen 73.

The Nearings are lactovegetarians. Their diet is 50 percent fruit, 35 percent vegetables, 10 percent protein and starch, and 5 percent fat. No candy, tea, coffee, alcohol, soft drinks, pastry or tobacco is used. When a sweetener is desired, honey is preferred, and a festive occasion may include ice cream. Food is often served raw. Otherwise, it is lightly steamed, boiled, or baked and served at room temperature in wooden utensils which are easy to clean and prevent any metallic poisoning. Most of the food comes from their own gardens, where synthetic chemicals and artificial substances of any kind are banned. Although they used animal manure in Vermont, in Maine they have used only "green compost." This practice is based on their moral premise that no living creature should exploit another and on the dietary belief that animal products are harmful to humans. Scott also likes to say that keeping animals is a chore and would make the travel he and his wife thrive on far more difficult.

Much of the Nearings' leisure time at home is spent in studying and writing. Some of their books are published through commercial houses, but others come out under their own imprint, which means they must oversee typesetting, printing, and a small mail-order operation. They travel a great deal to gather new experiences and to teach in various settings, including universities, fairs, and international health congresses. Other parts of their non-bread-labor time are devoted to local social activities, such as a town meeting or a musical evening at home. New ideas and projects continue to be the manna of their lives. After a visit to China, Scott undertook to adapt some of the agricultural techniques he saw there to his Maine garden. He plans to write a book on longevity, which would be a good companion to the book he wrote with Helen on how to build a low-cost greenhouse that makes it possible to have year-round gardens in climates as cold as Maine. A film made in 1978 shows Scott explaining his ideas with consistent wit and humor,[19] and a photo story a year later in *The New York Times* identified him as the oldest author at that year's major book fair. Retirement, to say the least, has never been part of the Nearing agenda.

A fuller review of the scope of Nearing's thought or that of Cornaro or of the 3 long-living physicians is not appropriate here. What is so remarkable about them is their passionate involvement with life for all of their considerable years. Yet there are many tens of thousands of others living just as vigorously who have become part of the anonymous legacy of history, the marvel of their lives known only to a few close associates and relatives.

Many interesting examples of longevous lives come to attention only through flukes. In the early 1970s, for instance, a video team interested in an unusual angle on black history discovered Mrs. Lula Sadler Craig, age 101, living on the Colorado prairie with her daughter and sister.[20] The crew filmed her reminiscing about black pioneers in the Old West, and covered a reunion in which hundreds of the matriarch's descendants converged to celebrate her 102nd birthday. Among the neighbors who dropped by to congratulate her was a centenarian cattle rancher. Similarly, Sula Benet, writing about the Soviet Union, mentions parenthetically stories about her friend Arthur "Chammy" Spurling, age 102, whom she met on vacations on Cranberry Island off the coast of Maine.[21] *The New York Times* of July 11, 1978, printed a photograph of Julius Kahn, age 99 years and 9 months, placing a kiss on the cheek of his wife, Della, at her 100th-birthday party. Later in the year the public relations department of American Telephone & Telegraph announced that its oldest known stockholder was Dolly Warren, age 106, who was still living in her own home in Washington, D.C. In

1979, the New York metropolitan newspapers wrote of Dr. Walter Pannell, who had been born July 31, 1879, yet was still walking to work and seeing patients at his East Orange, New Jersey, office. Dr. Pannell, now over 100, had been practicing medicine for seventy-five years.[22]

No selective list, however, long, could begin to do justice to more than a fraction of the octogenarians, nonagenarians, and centenarians who have lived their final years with gusto. The samplings only serve as indications of the tremendous range of creativity, satisfaction, and adventure that can be savored at an advanced age. They are the best riposte to those who protest, "Why would anyone want to live to be a hundred?"

The biographies of long-living persons also give a realistic measurement of the outer limits of human life. With the possible exception of Shigechiyo Izumi, there is no compelling evidence that anyone has ever lived more than 114 years. Given that the vast percentage of the world's population born previous to the twentieth century is undocumented, it is not unreasonable to believe that some persons may have lived longer than Izumi or Filkins, but it is unlikely that their number is large. To have even one individual living to the age of 117, there would have to be a cluster at 116 as well as additions to all the ranks between 110 and 115. It is highly improbable that such a special group would have been "missed" in the available histories, biographies, and oral traditions that can be drawn on. A human life-span of approximately 115 to 120 years is compatible with current biological assessments of the capacities of the vital parts of the human body. None of these appear to be programmed to wear out before a hundred years, but many approach minimal efficiency shortly thereafter.[23]

For the purpose of life extension, determining just how far beyond 114 humans might live without artificial means is less critical than addressing the three-decade gap between the average life-span in developed nations and the life-span possible if there is no premature aging. By examining the lives of people who have actually lived through all or most of that gap, often with brilliance and vigor, it has been possible to identify a number of factors concerning physical activity, diet, and attitude. The longevity agenda that follows takes up each component in detail and provides ways of incorporating prolongevous habits into a contemporary life-style. The expectation is that the agenda can greatly increase the prospects of reaching 85 with the kind of health momentum needed to make a 100th birthday a plausible goal.

Part Two

THE LONGEVITY AGENDA

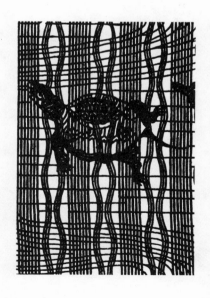

8

DOCTOR TWO LEGS

I have two doctors, my left leg and
my right. When body and mind are
out of gear (and those twin parts of
me live at such close quarters that
the one always catches melancholy
from the other), I know that I shall
have only to call in my two doctors
and I shall be well again.

—*Sir George Macaulay Trevelyan*

Strenuous physical activity throughout the course of life is
the most common thread in the biographies of longevous
people. Nonetheless, every winter individuals will die from
the exertion of shoveling snow, and every summer tennis
players and golfers contribute a fair percentage of heart-attack
and heat-stroke victims. In the United States, many high
school athletes will develop degenerative diseases by mid-
life, and as a group, male professional athletes have life-spans
below the national averages. These paradoxes demonstrate
that physical exercise, perhaps the single most important
item in the longevity agenda, can be a cruel double-edged
sword that must be approached as objectively as one approaches the age claims of supercentenarians.

The routines that best fulfill prolongevous criteria are
built around the most natural movements of the body. To
have a prolongevous effect, these movements must promote

oxygen efficiency, skeletal durability, and muscular strength without jeopardizing the body with unnecessary strain or tension. They must be congenial enough to become part of everyday life and pursuable in some variation to the hundredth year and beyond. The five common exercises that meet these criteria, if done properly, are walking, hiking, cross-country skiing, jogging, and swimming.

Walking is tops because it can be accommodated to the daily routine with the least disruption, is the safest form of exercise, requires no special equipment or physical setting, and can be undertaken for hours on end with the body gaining power continuously. In some cultures it is normal to walk in excess of 20 miles a day, and Native Americans such as the Apache could walk 40 to 50 miles a day through the desert without ill effects. Being completely natural to the body, walking is a movement that can be carried on at any age, and it is the exercise overwhelmingly preferred by people over 70.[1] Most persons who reach their 100th year have literally walked most of the way.

Hiking may be thought of as walking in nature. Once basic conditioning of the body has taken place, the activity may go on for hours without fatigue. Whether with a backpack for overnight camping or just a knapsack for snacks, hiking, thanks to the challenge of terrain and the need to climb or scramble over rocks, accelerates the buildup of muscular strength and overall vigor. It is slightly less safe than walking because of the greater possibility of falling or becoming exhausted, but limiting hiking to well-marked nature trails greatly reduces even these minor risks.

Cross-country skiing is a kind of hiking on snow. While it does not have the climbing factor that hiking does, it burns even more calories, because of the equipment involved and the winter temperatures, and is an excellent muscle builder. The sport is extremely popular in Scandinavia, a region with some of the longest average life-spans found anywhere in the world; and a study of 396 Finnish champion endurance skiers born between 1845 and 1910 revealed that they outlived their long-living fellow citizens by from five to seven years.[2]

The major advantage of jogging over hiking or walking is that it can achieve the same benefits in a shorter space of time. Another attraction is that jogging is easily adapted to an urban setting and a crowded daily schedule. Using only earth or grass surfaces is an important longevity consideration, as a hard surface such as concrete may promote long-term wear-and-tear factors in sensitive parts of the body. But most injuries arising from walking or running activities are associated with participation in marathon or speed-racing events, both of which will be dealt with shortly.

Swimming is the only one of the top five exercises that is not an obvious variation of walking. Any stroke is pro-longevously acceptable as long as the swimming is continued for an hour. The major drawback is that doing laps in a pool or swimming back and forth across the same lake may become tedious as a daily activity. More often than not, swimming is an occasional or seasonal alternative for one of the other top four. Its chief advantage is that by virtue of working every muscle in the body, it is unbeatable for overall toning.

Except for the disadvantage that they work only parts of the body, other activities of outstanding merit include cycling, sawing, digging, and rowing. Most people building an exercise agenda will find that a variety of activities is preferable to concentrating on just one or two. The standard to follow is that the number of calories burned per hour should be between 400 and 500, or the amount burned by walking from 4 to 5 miles in an hour. This output must be achieved over the whole hour, with only minor fluctuations from minute to minute. Reaching the same or even higher total caloric output with short bursts of energy followed by rest periods does not have the same prolongevous effect, any more than does carrying out a relatively lazy 200-calorie activity for two hours. The range of 400 to 500 calories an hour also brings about prolongevous conditioning of the heart by making it work at a rate of from 70 to 90 percent of its maximum capacity.

Before proceeding to make selections based on the charts and considerations that follow, it is important to understand what conditioning means in relationship to various biological processes. The maintenance and strengthening effect of conditioning is most readily observed in the respiratory and cardiovascular systems. Forcing the lungs to work strenuously over a protracted period of time is the only way to maintain their overall capacity to pull in the oxygen essential for all bodily functions. The vital capacity of the lungs of sedentary people diminishes in direct proportion to their sloth, progressively causing them to feel short-winded or out of breath with the slightest exertion. By contrast, the lungs of active people will show no significant decline over many decades. The same exercises also strengthen the muscles around the lungs so that the amount of oxygen available on short notice can be greatly increased, doubling the advantage vis-à-vis the inactive. Meanwhile, the arterial system which carries the oxygen to waiting cells and organs is being assisted. The arteries expand and are kept junk-free by the burning off of waste products, which otherwise might accumulate as dangerous plaque. Simultaneously with this housekeeping, new vessels are being created. Some of them will go around blockages that have already formed, and others will improve circulation in neglected parts of the body. These new passages take some time to construct and come into play only as complete networks, thereby accounting for the sudden surge of strength an individual will feel after being on a program for a few weeks.

The net result of the improvement of the cardiorespiratory system is that every cell and organ of the body operates at increased efficiency. The "high" often reported by joggers is the immediate invigorating impact of oxygen-rich blood on the brain cells, while the feeling of power is partly related to the impact of oxygen on the vital organs. A major long-range anti-wear-and-tear dividend is that the conditioned heart at rest needs to beat less rapidly in order to maintain the body's support systems. Furthermore, as various materials can be taken from and added to the bloodstream with reduced effort, the blood itself flows at lower pressure, reducing dangers that could come from hypertension. The heart, having become fully oxygenated, is not likely to be prone to damage from fibrillation, a frequent cause of heart attacks.

Equally dramatic changes occur in the muscular and skeletal systems. New muscles are created, and old muscle tissue, instead of hanging free of the skeletal frame as happens in inactive people, remains taut. Thanks to the rhythmic patterns of movement, the muscles become lithe and elongated, giving the body the wiry strength characteristic of the longevous. The same movements stimulate bone marrow, so that the density of bone is either maintained or increased. Muscles in the digestive tract are also stimulated, which aids evacuation and has an overall relaxing effect. Secondary benefits include input into the regulation of sleep, control of appetite, prevention of minor aches, discouragement of varicose veins, tightening of loose skin, and, of course, burning of stored fat.

Such gains, it must be stressed, occur only when the activity takes place over an extended period without being carried to the point of fatigue. The rhythmic factor is just as crucial. Without it, stress, jolting, and tension can have harmful consequences for organs, muscles, ligaments, nerves, and other bodily components. Prolongevous activities must not be confused with somewhat similar activities which may be fun to do but are either neutral or negative in their longevous effects. Usually, these are sports or exercises that emphasize a single aspect of the body such as form, stamina, coordination, speed, or strength. Frequently, they involve dubious diets, supplements, and movements. Because the aims are usually linked to athletic competition or aesthetic ideals rather than overall health, they may be considered longevity sidetracks. Examining a few of them helps to define what is prolongevously desirable and what is not.

The muscle-building sidetrack. Working any particular group of muscles will stimulate their growth. Hardening of the abdomen may be accomplished through multiple sit-ups, and building biceps can be accomplished by lifting weights. The effects on longevity of this kind of caloric output are minimal and in some instances harmful. In order to lift extraordinarily heavy weights, the lifter must have layers and layers of fat to support the overdeveloped muscle, and the jerking motions involved in the actual lifting place sudden and possibly traumatic demands upon the heart. Muscle can become so unnaturally developed that the normal functioning of the joints and connective tissues is prevented. Professional muscle men do not enjoy long life-spans, and manipulating any muscle group beyond the point needed for survival activities may be a gross distortion of bodily design. What constitutes "the body beautiful" is a matter of aesthetic taste. Bulging muscles are no more inherently desirable than necks stretched by rows of metal braces or feet withered through binding.

The skill sidetrack. Ballet students undergo extremely long and physically arduous training programs. Their caloric output is high and they achieve incredible muscular control, yet because of the stop-start nature of the dancing and extreme stress on various parts of the anatomy, ballet dancers have no longevous advantages. Those fascinated by the challenge of golfing or bowling are in a related category. They may be having a good time, but the longevous impact of hours of play is not much greater than that for stationary sports like skeet shooting, billiards, or shuffleboard. More strenuous games like tennis, handball, and squash may develop excellent eye-and-hand coordination as well as other skills, but the stop-start pattern of play, the jerking movements, and the fatigue induced by playing in the sun or in stuffy enclosures neutralize most systemic benefits. Many other activities have similar positive-and-negative pairings which are in such close balance that they do not hold prolongevous interest; but sports with heavy body contact should be avoided altogether. Bruises, sprains, and fractures are only the most visible antilongevous dangers. An indication of how antithetical such sports may be to long life is that the average life-spans of male professional boxers and football players in the United States are below those of heavy smokers and from ten to fifteen years less than those of the average male.

The stamina sidetrack. Many activities, such as jogging, swimming, dancing, and cycling, that are prolongevous when done for limited periods of time become of dubious or negative value when extended into a marathon phase. Even walking can be carried to excess. The most popular marathon walking events are to walk 100 miles in one day or to walk 1 mile for one thousand consecutive hours, with part of each hour given to sleep or rest. The problem with these and other marathon exploits is that the longer the body is worked, the closer it will come to a fatigue point at which dangers from injury and stress begin to overcome the health benefits. Signs of this changeover from prolongevous to neutral to antilongevous effects include dehydration and inflammation of the joints, but the most unmistakable one is the period of general collapse which occurs at the conclusion of an event like the Boston Marathon or a six-day bicycle race. Depending on the exact circumstances and the condition of the competitor, the time needed for recuperation may last from several hours to days to weeks. World-record seekers in marathon events often need as many months to recover from their feats as were required to train for them.[3] This pattern bears little resemblance to prolongevous activities, which should leave the individual with an immediate sense of well-being and provide the body with greater strength for the following day's routines.

The speed sidetrack. Running very rapidly over a short course or swimming several laps at top speed is debilitating.

Projecting the minute-by-minute caloric output to see what would be expended over an hour is illusory, for the pace could never be maintained. Rather than promoting the kind of steady oxygen efficiency that is of benefit in daily life, racing is a severe test which very swiftly draws extraordinary amounts of oxygen from the lungs. This sudden oxygen withdrawal is so enormous that the stress can trigger a heart attack. This rarely occurs in athletes who have trained methodically for racing competition and who understand their capacities, but even they must sit quietly, gulping down fresh oxygen to restore their strength as soon as the event is completed. The dangers of oxygen depletion can be fatal for otherwise sedentary people who suddenly have the urge to dance all night, shovel snow, or take part in a game of touch football. Another danger from speed events is that they may put severe pressure on the joints and organs because of the momentum involved. This drawback is multiplied when leaping or jumping is involved.

People caught up in longevity sidetracks usually begin to alter their diet so that it may better support their exercises. This often means a misplaced faith in animal protein, mineral supplements, megavitamin intake, and sugar. Even when this is not the case, the diet is deflected from the goal of supporting overall health to supporting a peculiar activity, such as swimming across the English Channel or lifting 200 pounds above one's head. The prolongevous never alter their diet in this manner. To put it more positively: the normal prolongevous diet also is the best diet for prolongevous exercises.

Other difficulties that may arise from sidetracking are the stresses resulting from distorting the daily schedule to fit in more and more exercise time and those created by trying to meet steadily rising performance expectations. Someone arising in the dawn to get in a few extra miles in preparation for a marathon or the swimmer constantly competing with a stopwatch is not on a prolongevous wavelength.

Most long-living people incorporate strenuous activities

into their habitual routines to the highest degree possible, have regular daily patterns, and monitor their health and exercise informally. Without falling into the rigidity of those caught up in longevity sidetracks, anyone embarking on a longevity agenda should check bodily responses more systematically than most longevous people have; they, after all, did not necessarily *plan* to be longevous. At the outset of a program it is wise to get blood-pressure, heart-efficiency, and cholesterol/triglyceride readings at a doctor's office. During the first year or so of the program, keeping track of these on a semiannual basis is useful. Once desired levels have been reached, the checkups can be extended to once every two or three years without any harm. There also is an extremely simple, cheap, and reliable measurement of the body's longevity potential which can be made at any time. That measure is total body weight.

Every longevity study cited so far has noted the spare somatype of the longevous, and it is axiomatic that in the animal world long life and restricted but wholesome diets go hand in hand. These observations find startling statistical confirmation in records compiled by various life-insurance companies in the United States. The companies keep track of the weight of their clients at the time of death. Their analysis, which is crucial to the decision making of multi-million-dollar enterprises, shows that it is almost impossible to be too lean. As long as one follows a prolongevous diet and as long as prolongevous exercises are part of daily life, light body weight provides one of the most reliable predictors of longevity at any given age. About the only exceptions are people who suffer from diseases and those who control their weight exclusively through diet. Obese persons are virtually precluded from longevity. A few overweight individuals, most of whom have become heavy relatively late in life, may be seen at age 90, but almost none will survive past 95. The operating principle is not that low body weight will produce longevity, but that longevous life-styles will produce low body weight.

Longevously desirable body weights are much lower than those popularly associated with good health. An impressive illustration of this is a chart created by the Metropolitan Life Insurance Company but based on the mortality statistics of 4 million clients of various such companies. It shows that the most longevous body weight for a man of 6 feet having a medium body frame is between 150 and 167 pounds. The findings in this chart, which are based on death from all causes, including accidents, indicate that from a longevous standpoint, well over 85 percent of all Americans are overweight. The excess fat in the 1970s ran to about 5 billion pounds.

DESIRABLE WEIGHTS[4]

Ages 25 and Over

HEIGHT (WITHOUT SHOES)	WEIGHT WITHOUT CLOTHING (POUNDS)		
	SMALL FRAME	MEDIUM FRAME	LARGE FRAME
MEN			
5 ft. 1 in.	104–112	110–121	118–133
5 ft. 2 in.	107–115	113–125	121–136
5 ft. 3 in.	110–118	116–128	124–140
5 ft. 4 in.	113–121	119–131	127–144
5 ft. 5 in.	116–125	122–135	130–148
5 ft. 6 in.	120–129	126–139	134–153
5 ft. 7 in.	124–133	130–144	139–158
5 ft. 8 in.	128–137	134–148	143–162
5 ft. 9 in.	132–142	138–152	147–166
5 ft. 10 in.	136–146	142–157	151–171
5 ft. 11 in.	140–150	146–162	156–176
6 ft.	144–154	150–167	160–181
6 ft. 1 in.	148–159	154–172	165–186
6 ft. 2 in.	152–163	159–177	170–191
6 ft. 3 in.	156–167	164–182	174–196

WOMEN

4 ft. 8 in.	87–93	91–102	99–114
4 ft. 9 in.	89–96	93–105	101–117
4 ft. 10 in.	91–99	96–108	104–120
4 ft. 11 in.	94–102	99–111	107–123
5 ft.	97–105	102–114	110–126
5 ft. 1 in.	100–108	105–117	113–129
5 ft. 2 in.	103–111	108–121	116–133
5 ft. 3 in.	106–114	111–125	120–137
5 ft. 4 in.	109–118	115–130	124–141
5 ft. 5 in.	113–122	119–134	128–145
5 ft. 6 in.	117–126	123–138	132–149
5 ft. 7 in.	121–130	127–142	136–153
5 ft. 8 in.	125–135	131–146	140–158
5 ft. 9 in.	129–139	135–150	144–163
5 ft. 10 in.	133–143	139–154	148–168

For weights with ordinary indoor clothing, add 5 pounds for women and 8 pounds for men to the above figures.

While the extent of the overweight problem may be surprising, its existence is not. Concern with excess poundage has long produced a torrent of books touting one more new system of weight reduction. Most of these methods are doomed to long-term failure because they are not concerned with overall life-styles. It has taken years for the overweight body to reach whatever dimension it has attained. Under the chin, around the belly, and in every nook of the body, there are veritable fat cities making constant demands upon the feeding, policing, and sewage systems of the body. Attempts to tear down the fat cities in a crash program further clog all vital networks, throwing the body into confusion and stressing the organism more than the stored fat had. The weakness, fatigue, and headaches experienced by people on trick or starvation diets are the body groaning under its ordeal. Many diets increase these dangers by encouraging potentially dangerous chemical reactions within the body. In place of this kind of chaos, the fat cities need to be torn down methodically, with the muscles rebuilt and the body toned as an integral part of the process. The answer lies in prolongevous exercise.

If one's present diet is maintaining rather than increasing total body weight, adding one hour of brisk walking to a daily schedule will burn off 400 calories a day, 2,800 a week, 1,200 a month, and 145,000 a year. Even when eating remains absolutely the same, this works out to a loss of more than 3 pounds a month and approximately 40 pounds a year—more than most people will lose on conventional weight-loss programs. While slimming down to the weights found in the insurance-company charts could take longer than a year, improvement in appearance begins in a matter of months and is dramatic by the end of the first year. The likelihood is that reduction will be faster the more overweight an individual is and slower the more closely exercise and diet, caloric output and caloric intake approach a dynamic balance. The best longevous weight would be at the lower end of the weight spectrum found in the life-insurance charts. Once at that weight, one could judge whether loss of another 5 to 10 pounds might make the body even stronger, but that is a matter of fine tuning highly dependent upon individual needs. Those who require muscle power in their work are likely to be heavier than those who work at desks.

The pace of weight reduction can always be accelerated by lowering caloric intake or by increasing exercise time, but under no circumstances should weight loss become yet another sidetrack. Internal body-management systems will gradually reshape the body along the lines most natural for the particular individual. The quickest spur to this process will come from walking or swimming, the exercises that provide gentle but constant toning of the muscles and skin. In this regard, even short walks of fifteen minutes to half an hour can be beneficial. On the other hand, motorized exercise machines are worthless for body rebuilding, and machines that stimulate the body with rollers or belts may cause internal bruises and other damage. Saunas, steam baths, and massages have a relaxing effect, but do not lead to weight loss or body shaping. Almost all schemes for spot reduction are futile, because when seeking energy the body takes fat from all cells, not just from those in the area immediately agitated.

Before undertaking any exercise agenda, individuals generally are better off consulting a physician to see if they have any ailments that might influence the kind of exercise they should include. But the program proper will begin with the bathroom scale. For a period of from a week to ten days, an individual should take his or her weight first thing in the morning and sometime late in the afternoon or early evening. There will be a fluctuation of some 5 to 6 pounds, which reflects consumption of water, particular menus, and other variables. Even after weight reduction begins, no one should ever expect a steadily declining curve. Instead, as with an ailing stock market in the course of a long downward trend, there will be unexpected highs and plateaus. Over a period of a month, however, a fluctuation that begins in the 155–160 range should go down to 153–159 and then proceed in the following months to 152–158 and so forth. Some individuals may prefer to continue the once-or twice-daily weight watching, living through the drops, plateaus, and highs, while others will be happier on a weekly or biweekly schedule. It makes no difference as long as the average weekly loss is no less than 1 pound and no more than 5. Below this level one is too close to just maintaining weight, and over it, the pace is likely to be too fast to maintain on a long-range basis without a feeling of weakness, discomfort, or sacrifice.

During the same week that people record their weight, they should determine how many miles they cover in a typical day. A simple method for doing this is to purchase a pedometer of the kind worn by hikers and to attach it to a belt or pocket. A prolongevous life-style should average about 10 miles a day over a week's time. Most Americans will find that their total comes to less than 3. Gradually closing the gap between their present exercise output and 10 provides the vast majority of people with an individual exercise goal. This does not mean they need to spend the rest of their lives strapped to a pedometer, only how many 4-to 5-mile walks or their equivalents should be considered. For example, if the total average daily mileage is 3, then one hour of walking or jogging would bring the total to over 7. Another way of addressing the 10-mile goal without the use of the pedometer is to put two hours of walking into the daily schedule. One hour should be continuous, but the other could be divided into two half-hour segments. The pace must be brisk, from 3.5 to 5 miles per hour.

Occasionally there may be daily routines that provide the 10-miles-a-day average without producing the desired somatype. This may be the result of the stop-and-start nature of work or, as is the case with many manual workers, of too much caloric intake. A possible solution is to shift more attention to diet control than is required of those still struggling with the problem of inactivity. More exercise also should be considered no matter how rigorous the workday seems on the surface. People in this situation, like those just beginning to become physically active, need to be aware of false fatigue. At the early stages of building a longevous body, it may take some will power to add another hour of walking. Later on, the same individual will find that he or she is uncomfortable when forced into idleness.

Scattering prolongevous activities throughout the daily and weekly schedule is the surest way of getting up to a 10-mile daily average that can be maintained for a lifetime. An excellent starting point is transportation. Those living within 5 miles of their place of employment could walk or ride a bike instead of taking motorized transportation. The suburban pattern in which one spouse regularly drives the other to the train depot could be replaced by having the commuting spouse walk or bike to the station whenever weather permits. In the city, one could get into the habit of getting off public transportation a few blocks early in order to walk the remaining distance or, if feasible, walking from a point where transfers are usually made. An advantage of the latter is that overall time may come out about the same, as part or all of the period formerly spent waiting is spent walking. Those who work in office buildings might forgo the elevator and climb stairs. Similar additions of walking can be made at lunchtime and after work, especially for shopping that does not require carrying heavy loads. The short car hop to the neighborhood store is another expendable. However brief the walk, it provides more stimulation than sitting in an automobile.

Within the household itself, many tasks that must be done anyway can be reprogrammed for longevity value. Mopping, sweeping, and waxing become prolongevous when they are done at a brisk tempo. From one-half to one full hour of any of them or a combination is the equivalent of walking for the same period. Once the body has gotten some conditioning, mowing the lawn twice a week with a hand mower can take the place of once-a-week mowing with a power machine. In the country, sawing wood with a hand tool or splitting logs is unbeatable. Whatever the household task, if it can be done vigorously and continuously with fluid motions it becomes beneficial. Transformation of essential labor in this manner has particular psychological comforts for those who do not enjoy formal exercise or who consider it frivolous.

The time normally spent on an evening of entertainment can be rendered prolongevous by a subtle shift of emphasis. Dancing, which is not normally thought of in terms of health, is an excellent prolongevous activity whether it takes the form of ballroom, folk, or free-form styles. The only drawback is that some dancing environments are filled with smoke or are quite noisy. For instance, contemporary discotheques with their brain-boggling flashing lights and over-amplified music are longevity chambers of horror.

In the summer, a day at the beach could involve an hour of swimming and long walks in the surf, but except for their social function, casual beach games like volleyball are not particularly invigorating. Watercraft of preference are any that require muscle power instead of motors or wind. On the shore or in the water, there should be as little cooking of the skin as possible. Tanning is a defense response of the body to the attack of the sun's ultraviolet rays. Consciously seeking a deep tan simply accelerates the aging of the skin and increases the risk of cancer. A far better strategy is to accept whatever sun is natural to the situation. Best of all, one should keep exposure to a minimum. In a park setting, time can be set aside for walking, horseback riding, or roller skating. Longevously neutral sports like golf can be improved upon if people pass up carts and caddies and carry their own clubs. Even a card game at a sprawling retirement condominium offers a longevity opening if players walk to the center instead of riding.

In winter, the best choice is cross-country skiing, but ice skating, sledding, and tobogganing are good too. The benefits of sledding and tobogganing, of course, are not in the slide down but in the climb to the top of the hill. If mechanized means are used for this, their longevous advantage is lost. Downhill skiing flunks out on this score, and it can easily abuse the body with its various jolting and straining movements. Hockey is almost as antilongevous as football because of the body checking involved. Snowmobiles are neutral at best.

Vacations extend all of the recreational possibilities into longer time frames and provide opportunities for extended camping-hiking trips. Especially in the United States, where there is natural splendor available everywhere, pursuit of longevity becomes a thrilling aesthetic experience in which the only hardship is the necessity of returning to the mundane world. Hiking, biking, and cross-country skiing all provide an excellent focus for activist holidays and weekends. Even those who prefer relatively effortless hunting or fishing vacations can improve them. Game that must be stalked can be substituted for prey that is waited for. Anglers can row rather than motor into the middle of the lake, and trout enthusiasts can get out of the stream for an occasional walk through the woods. People who center vacations on visits to urban centers can do the town on foot as much as possible. They will see more, get a better sense of the place's real ambiance, and perhaps save a little money. Whatever the vacation, staying on one's feet, not off them, is the surest way to get the relaxation holidays are designed for.

Back at the workplace, any procedures requiring physical movement should be bunched up into continuous segments for the longevity bonus. Those who work at desk jobs will find that if they get up at least once every hour to stretch and move about, they will become more clearheaded and will feel much more energetic. Although exercise time and gym facilities as fringe benefits are a new concept, asking for them in a labor negotiation is not out of the question. Major corporations like Kimberly-Clark have found that providing a full-scale gym for clerical, manual, and managerial workers to use at various times during the day raises productivity and cuts into the number of days lost to illness. Even in the most conventional setups, there are likely to be missed opportunities for prolongevous activities both during the work and afterward. Schoolteachers who hurry home after a tough day to relax with a cigarette, martini, or coffee would be better off using their school gym for an hour.

The relaxing effect of exercise is particularly significant in a nation in which tension is a major health complaint. A number of tests have pitted walking against the most common tranquilizers and other drugs to see which relaxant is the more effective in lowering blood pressure, relieving nervous tension, and combating tightened muscles. Walks of approximately fifteen minutes proved more effective in both the short and long term, even without factoring in possible side effects from chronic use of medication. This principle was understood in ancient Greece, where Aristotle, among others, taught that people should walk as they carried on a discourse or attempted to think out a problem. A more familiar instance is the expectant father walking off his anxiety by pacing outside a delivery room.

A home garden, with its multiple demands on all parts of the body, scores extremely well on the longevity scale. When briskly done, movements like hoeing, digging, and raking for an hour at a time are equivalent or superior to jogging. Bending to pull weeds, staking up plants, tugging at sacks of manure, and other strenuous chores all tote up numerous pluses for the musculoskeletal system. More so than most activities, gardening can expand into a multi-hour exertion with little sense of time imposition or hardship. The ultimate production of food or flowers provides a unique and satisfying reward for the energy expended.

A certain personality type will be more comfortable with a formal set of exercise routines and a system to measure bodily response. Such individuals can develop their own routines using tables found in the Canadian Air Force program,[5] the aerobic system of Kenneth Cooper,[6] or the exercise mode of the Pritikin Plan.[7] The major caution in dealing with these systems is that they are aimed primarily at promoting cardiovascular health rather than longevity per se. As such, they are somewhat less sensitive to long-term wear-and-tear problems than they should be. As the prolongevous person wants to be walking fast and hard at age 90, the effects of exercises on ankles, tendons, bones, ligaments, and joints are major considerations. Plans of the kind cited also have a tendency to demand less in terms of time commitment than is really needed to pile up longevity gains. This is particularly true of the Canadian plan.

The risk of unnecessary wear and tear once more places walking in the longevity spotlight. Given a choice between running in place and taking a walk, the walk is superior on at least three counts. First, it is much easier to upgrade to a walking speed of 4 miles an hour than it is to reach the equivalent by running in place. Second, natural movements are always easier and more benevolent for the body than artificial ones. People who run in place frequently experience stiffness or cramps in their legs. Third, when getting close to a walking pace of 5 miles an hour, the body usually yearns to set off into a jog, and a walk/jog pattern may develop. Increasing the speed, however, is less important than continuing the activity for at least an hour. Those with conservative temperaments should not think of this behavior as a newfangled health craze. It is a modern reassertion of the old American habit of a daily constitutional. President Harry S. Truman was an avid walker whose brisk gait often left reporters panting. When still a senator, Truman had noted that his fellow senators were dying of heart disease at an alarming rate. He asked a doctor what preventive measure he should take and was told to start walking.

Particular exercises may be appealing because of the time involved. Ten minutes of skipping rope in the style of a professional boxer can equal an hour of walking. Yet it is not really a good regular prolongevous exercise because of possible jolting of the body, oxygen depletion, and stressing of joints. When faced with exercise choices, one is best advised to be on the cautious side at all times, and if warm-ups are required, they should never be dismissed as unnecessary. It is also important to bear in mind that one doesn't have to sweat to get longevity benefits. Walking a mile burns up about as many calories as jogging does; it just takes longer.

Many games and activities are fun to do even though they are not particularly prolongevous. As long as they are not harmful, there is no reason to give them up. But when promoting longevity is the goal, the activities in the following tables are decidedly superior. The indicated caloric outputs are approximations subject to individual factors, such as personal weight, terrain, and speed. All activities are calculated on a one-hour basis.

The following activities are good for those beginning a program or as supplements to more strenuous activities. They expend from 300 to 350 calories an hour.

- Walking from 2 to 3.5 miles per hour.
- Cycling from 5 to 8 miles per hour.
- Ice- or roller-skating slowly, but with little coasting.

- Moderately paced housekeeping like cleaning, mopping, vacuuming, waxing, and making beds.
- Mowing the lawn with a hand mower.
- Dancing slowly.

The following activities should be the center of most programs. They expend from 350 to 500 calories an hour.

- Walking or jogging or walk/jogging from 3.5 to 5 miles per hour.
- Cycling from 8 to 11 miles per hour.
- Hiking from 3 to 5 miles per hour.
- Cross-country skiing from 3 to 5 miles per hour.
- Swimming at a moderate speed.
- Ice- or roller-skating rapidly.
- Vigorously paced housekeeping.
- Dancing strenuously.
- Digging, hoeing, or raking.
- Shoveling snow.
- Splitting logs or sawing wood.
- Rowing slowly.

The following activities should be done only by those who are in condition. They expend over 500 calories an hour.

- Walking more than 5 miles per hour on an incline.
- Jogging more than 5.5 miles per hour.
- Hiking in rugged terrain.
- Vigorous cross-country skiing.
- Vigorous swimming.
- Cycling over 13 miles per hour.
- Rowing rapidly.
- Horseback riding at a gallop.
- Walking up and down stairs.

No exercise agenda, whatever its particulars, should be rigid. While the program is best followed each day, when the weather is uncooperative or when the air quality is adverse, a shift to indoor activities or even inactivity may be best. The same holds true when walking or running can be done only by the side of busy motorways. There's no longevity gain in having the lungs inhale large amounts of poisoned air which the body will have to contend with for hours. There also is no cause for alarm if any given day falls into a series of events that does not allow the usual exercise. Many people find that an on-day/off-day pattern accommodates their bodies more efficiently. A physiological factor involved here is that muscle building involves tearing down old tissues, making a day of rest advisable if the workouts are strenuous. For this reason, body builders frequently manipulate different muscle groups on alternate days. If such a pattern seems advisable, then the off-day level may fall below 5 miles while the on-day goes to 15 or beyond. In any case, once the body has been conditioned, one or two days a week should have accelerated activity.

That age is no barrier to prolongevous exercise is demonstrated by the amazing athletic feats of many older people. In July, 1978, for example, Walter Poenisch, a 65-year-old retired baker from Ohio, completed a 33-hour nonstop swim from Havana, Cuba, to Little Duck Key, Florida, a distance of 125 miles. Poenisch had not taken up long-distance swimming until after age 50, and he undertook the marathon swim to publicize his concern for international friendship rather than to establish an athletic record. Because he used flippers during his swim, he could not qualify as a formal world-record holder.

Such was not the case for Dr. James Counsilman, who in September, 1979, at the age of 58, became the oldest person to swim the English Channel, making the crossing in thirteen hours. A year earlier, Ardath Evitt, age 74, became the oldest female ever to make a parachute jump. The oldest male is Bob Broadbere, age 85. Among remarkable walkers there is Dr. Barbara Moore, who in 1960, at the age of 56, walked 1,000 miles from northern Scotland to Land's End in Cornwall in 23 days. A month later she walked from San Francisco to New York City in 85 days. In 1976, Plennie Wingo, age 81,

walking *backward*, completed the 452 miles between Santa
Monica and San Francisco in 85 days. Edward Payson Weston
walked from New York City to San Francisco in 123 days at
the age of 71, and walked from New York City to Minneapolis in 56 days at the age of 75.

Interest in the physical performance of older people is so
recent that almost all running records for various age groups
date from the late 1970s and are constantly being broken. As
part of the running craze which swept the United States in
that decade, septuagenarians began to compete regularly in
what was called senior or masters competition. Records for
the eighth decade of life include runs of from 7 to 9 miles
within one hour's time, running 6 miles in times ranging
from 41 minutes to a little over 48, and running 1 mile in
times ranging from under 6 to under 7 minutes. Octogenarians have run in 100-, 200-, 400-, and 800-meter races
as well as in Olympic-length marathons. At age 91, Duncan
McClean set an age record in the 200-meter event of under 1
minute, and at age 93, he established an age record of 20.7
seconds for the 100 meters. Robert Willis, at age 90, was
clocked in the 9,800-meter marathon at 8:54.2. The most
durable nonagenarian runner, however, was Demetrios Iordanidis of Greece, who ran a 26.2-mile marathon race in 6
hours and 42 minutes at the age of 95. He returned three
years later, at age 98, to do it again, in a time of 7 hours and
33 minutes. Asked why he needed an extra hour the second
time, he quipped, "I was younger before."[8] Among his
prescriptions for long and robust life were no smoking, no
meat, drink milk, lots of walking, and no sex after age 85.

Running records for older women are less spectacular
than those for men because sexism makes it much more
socially difficult for senior women to train and compete
regularly. Nevertheless, there are many runners in their 60s
and 70s, and there are a few in their 80s. None is more
amazing than Eula Weaver, who holds records in the 800- and
1,500-meter events for an octogenarian female of ages 85, 86,
and 88. Her story is even more intriguing in that she was at

death's door during the decades of her late maturity. At age 67, Mrs. Weaver had suffered from angina; at age 75, she was hospitalized with heart disease; and at age 81, she suffered congestive heart failure. Her circulation at that time was so feeble that she had to wear gloves in the summer months to keep warm, and she was so weak that she could not walk more than a dozen feet without collapsing. Desperate to regain her health, Weaver put herself in the care of a longevity center operated by Nathan Pritikin. She began a program of gradual walk/jogging and shifted to a pro-longevous diet. In a year she was able to dispense with her medications. In two she would walk 3 miles at a time and could chalk up 10 miles a day on her stationary bicycle. In 1974 she began to set her running records. In 1979 she achieved her 90th birthday, to become a longevous person. Shortly thereafter Pritikin wrote that she ". . . is faithful to her diet, jogs one mile daily, lifts weights twice weekly, and feels fit as a fiddle."[9]

The prolongevous lesson to be drawn from these extraordinary exploits is that after conditioning of the body takes place, people in late maturity and beyond can demand active lives of themselves. Looking at a broad spectrum of time, the exercise program from ages 30 to 80 need not alter significantly, and after age 80, changes should be of degree, not kind. As for restrictions based upon sex, it is safe to say that the males should be able to keep up with the sturdier females as long as the usual precautions are taken against exercising to the point of fatigue or exhaustion.

When one is setting up an exercise agenda, a few points of reference should be kept in mind. Paramount is that one is not living in order to exercise well (much less to break physical records) but is exercising in order to live well. The slim, wiry prolongevous somatype is not to be acquired by obsessive efforts; it simply will follow from a combination of prolongevous dietary and exercise habits. The prolongevous exercises, characteristically rhythmic in nature and maintained for approximately an hour at a time, should be movements one likes to make, sees as valuable, and thinks of as easy. The activities should be planned to be done alone if need be, but group involvement can be strongly reinforcing. Activities should be noncompetitive for the most part, and skill in them a strictly secondary concern. Schedules must remain flexible, and as long as there is genuine movement toward reaching clearly defined goals, gradualism is the preferred speed of change. By far the best pattern is one in which a mixture of vigorous physical activities is an integral part of everyday life.

The exercise component of the longevity agenda constantly rebuilds and maintains the body, from its humblest cell to its most complex organ. Without this daily stimulation, the vital systems will decline far more rapidly than genetically programmed, bringing on premature aging and its fatal companion. Some benefits, such as light body weight, can be achieved through means such as diets and drugs, but the total positive impact on the system depends on exercise. Nothing can take its place. Exercise, in fact, will minimize the need for special diets, supplements, and medications. The key skill involved is a natural movement normally mastered by the end of the first year of life: walking.

9

FOOD AS FUEL

If we lived entirely on raw, fresh plant foods, as our ancestors did millions of years ago, there would be no need for concern about getting adequate amounts of the essential foods such as vitamins.

—*Linus Pauling*

The ceremonial importance of food is unarguable. Feasts are the centerpieces of many national holidays, and some foods have come to possess overriding patriotic significance. Enormous psychological investments are made in being excellent connoisseurs, cooks, and gourmets. Food often plays a symbolic role in religious rites or is thought to have curative or rejuvenating powers. When asked the secret of long life, centenarians often allude flippantly to food. A typical example is Mrs. May Lauchuck of Poughkeepsie, New York, age 104, who advised, "Take a teaspoonful of vodka laced with garlic twice a day"—a formula at odds with that of Signora Paolina Pichi of Borgonesia, Italy, also age 104, who recommended eating spaghetti three times a day. All of these mystifications of eating mask the essential reality that food is the fuel of the body. This being so, a prolongevous diet is one that furnishes the kind of fuel that permits the body to maintain its functions for as long as possible.

The major obstacle to determining a prolongevous diet is that there is so much biochemical individuality that no single diet can ever be ideally suited to every individual. Food that is excellent for one person may be harmful to another. The search for a prolongevous diet is further complicated by the incomplete state of our knowledge. It is still not certain what constitutes the optimal daily intake of the known essential nutrients, let alone essential nutrients not yet identified. Accordingly, attempts to limit eating to narrowly defined lists of prolongevous food are foolish and quite possibly hazardous. Only the general outline of a preferred diet can be projected. Pertinent to this task are the lifelong eating habits of the longevous, particularly centenarians.

The major characteristic of the diet of longevous people is low total caloric intake throughout life. Otherwise, the food eaten by the longevous is not greatly different from that consumed by the shorter-living population, with the exception that longevous people tend to eat far less meat. In terms of calories, the longevous have a daily intake of from 1,500 to 2,000 calories, as opposed to the average American intake of from 3,000 to 4,000. Moreover, whereas the typical American diet at the end of the twentieth century contains 40 to 45 percent fats, 15 to 20 percent proteins, and 35 to 45 percent carbohydrates (with the percentage of fats on the rise and the percentage of complex carbohydrates on the wane), the representative diet of the longevous contains about 10 to 15 percent fats, 10 to 15 percent proteins, and 70 to 80 percent carbohydrates (mainly complex).

In addition to using the diet of the longevous as a guideline in determining the optimal fuels, it is necessary to pay due respect to the design of the body, and specifically the design of the digestive system.[1] Moral considerations aside, such an appraisal discloses that the high proportion of meat found in most modern diets is inappropriate. To begin with, the human hand, without strong claws, is not well adapted to killing and dismembering other creatures. Instead, the fingers are wonderfully shaped for picking and pulling fruits, nuts, and vegetables. The teeth, similarly, are better designed to gnash vegetable matter than to tear flesh, the so-called canines being puny instruments for ripping when compared with those of undisputed carnivores. Further, human saliva, which breaks down food in the mouth, is alkaline, as in herbivores, containing ptyalin, an enzyme that predigests starch from plants. Farther along the digestive tract, the stomach, which can accommodate a dazzling variety of foods, still does not have the powerful kind of acids needed to deal with whole small game such as the freshly killed mouse that a cat's stomach handles perfunctorily.

The most dramatic indication of the noncarnivorous nature of the human digestive system is its overall length and shape. The digestive tract of a carnivore is usually three times the length of its torso, as measured from mouth to anus. This shortness allows for quick processing and rapid evacuation so that meat does not decay within the intestines and give off toxins. The human tract is about twelve times the length of the torso—four times as long as that of the carnivores and one-fourth longer than that of most herbivores. The human system has a very long convoluted small intestine followed by a large smoother one. Humans, like herbivores, drink by sucking rather than lapping, sweat through the skin rather than the tongue, and have alkaline urine. Taking secondary traits into account, the human system most closely resembles that of mammals, such as gorillas, which feed mainly on fruits, nuts, and grains. It is significant also that whereas carnivores are instinctively aroused by the smell of bleeding raw flesh and are indifferent to the aroma of ripe fruit, humans are not.

The most widely accepted resolution of these facts is to categorize the human species as omnivorous. Even if accurate, this classification would not indicate what percentage of the total diet meat should occupy. Anthropologists working with prehistoric skeletal remains have determined that originally humans were primarily fruit eaters and that after flesh entered the diet the ratio of plant food to meat was about 3 to

1—the reverse of the pattern in many contemporary diets. The gradual tilt to meat was a consequence of the improvement of hunting technology, the domestication of some animals, and the development of agriculture. Meat ceased to be a food of opportunity, and the range of plant food eaten dwindled considerably. However, the mere fact that meat eating is gastronomically possible and economically convenient does not make it desirable, especially if meat is treated as a staple.

All available studies indicate that exclusive or predominantly vegetarian diets result in longer average life-spans by from five to ten years. To be sure, some of these studies have used organized groups, such as the Seventh-Day Adventists, or informal movements, such as the grain-oriented macrobiotic advocates, in which there is tremendous social support for many prolongevous habits. This makes it impossible to credit the diet as the decisive factor; but even cautiously interpreted, the prolongevous findings indicate that nonmeat diets in no way retard long life, while leaving open the question of the degree of benefit.[2] Vegetarian groups have extremely low rates of hypertension, hyperglycemia, and hypoglycemia. Conversely, populations with the highest rates of beef intake have the highest rates of cancer, particularly of the breast and colon.

Because of their sensitivity to the nutritional value of food, vegetarians of choice enjoy another longevous benefit. They rightly believe that the less a food has been tampered with and the faster it arrives from the earth, the more nutritious it is. Most vegetarians, therefore, will try to live in situations in which they have access to garden-fresh vegetables and would consider the Abkhasian habit of eating freshly picked greens for breakfast a sensible one. Those who include cereals in their meals eat only whole grains, understanding that milling away the germ or seed robs the grain of its most nutritious part as well as its brownish hue.

The worldwide infatuation with white rice, white pasta, and white bread is one of the most absurd and tragic of human follies. Countless hours are wasted lowering the quality of food. In the United States, the devitalization of grain takes some bizarre twists. Commercial bakeries with national distribution will advertise that they have added a dozen or more vitamins to breads when in fact the overall processing actually has taken away many more nutrients than are returned. Some firms will use caramel coloring in their dough to make their products look like whole-grain loaves. The superiority of whole grains is so incontrovertible that anyone mildly interested in longevity should use them exclusively. The vitamin and mineral value of fresh vegetables and fruits is so widely appreciated that the same rule should apply whenever possible.

The most basic tampering with food is the cooking process. A diet nearest to that afforded by nature would concentrate on raw foods—nuts, seeds, greens, fruits, and berries. Food that must be prepared or softened will suffer the least nutritional loss if steamed, boiled, or baked, and the broth left over from steaming or boiling can be consumed as a soup to recover most of the loss. The form of cooking to be studiously avoided is frying. Whether frying oil begins as a saturate or an unsaturate, when heating commences the oil becomes saturated, and fat permeates the food. Vital elements like enzymes are destroyed by frying, and the food is made more difficult to digest, placing extra burdens on all parts of the digestive apparatus. Many otherwise excellent foods, such as the potato, are transformed into antilongevous junk when turned into French-fries or potato chips. By contrast, a baked potato, spared a butter-and-salt bath, is extremely nutritious and easy to digest.

The perennial debate about the advisability of dairy products to the diet has been given a new dimension by the controversy over the possible harm to the cardiovascular system by a high intake of cholesterol. Numerous vegetarians who abstain from dairy products on the ground that they are simply another form of unneeded animal exploitation point out that humans are the only known creatures to consume milk after infancy and that many adults cannot tolerate lactose. Other vegetarians respond that dairy products are rich in protein and contain many key nutrients such as calcium.[3] For them, the only danger is in excessive consumption. The matter cannot be resolved on strictly statistical grounds, as there are no studies comparing vegetarians who use no animal products of any kind with those who do. It should be emphasized that there is a strong moral dimension to the arguments of most of those who disapprove of using animal products and that spokespeople for that point of view make rather modest claims for the longevity benefit incurred. H. J. Dinshah, a leading vegetarian writer and publisher, who argues against exploiting any creature, believes that humans who do not eat flesh or flesh by-products can live in good health through their 80s but that few will surpass 100 years.[4]

Conflicting findings from various studies of the impact of high-cholesterol diets on health were clarified somewhat in the 1970s by explication of the effects of the two major types of cholesterol, high-density, or alpha, lipids and low-density, or beta, lipids. The latter are health culprits because they can attach to the arterial wall, where they often build up in sufficient quantity to cause blockage of the type treated by bypass surgery. High-density lipids, on the other hand, do not attach to arterial walls, but break down the beta lipids and help transport betas out of the body. Of longevous interest was the discovery that strenuous exercise stimulates bodily production of alpha cholesterol. Many of the previous studies which had shown no correlation between heart disease and high-cholesterol diets could be interpreted in a new light. The Masai people, for example, had long been cited as a group with excellent cardiovascular health in spite of the enormous amount of cholesterol in their diet. A possible explanation for this might be that the Masai walk up to 20 miles a day tending their herds.

The ratio of alpha lipids to betas in newborns is about 1 to 1, while in most adults it is 1 to 4. Moving downward from the adult range toward the level of newborns might be a good long-range goal, but it should not be pursued compulsively. Attempts to stimulate alpha production through medication or other artificial means is unwise, in that the long-term side effects may be harmful and some subdivisions within the alphas appear to be as harmful as excessive betas. The best longevity strategy is to maintain a low overall cholesterol level through the choice of natural foods. Any effort to lower the beta proportion also should be made through food selection or through prolongevous exercises of the kind already delineated.

Even discounting consideration of the alpha–beta subdivision, longevous people usually have much lower overall cholesterol levels than their shorter-lived fellow citizens. The old rule of thumb that a reading of 200 plus one's age is acceptable is a longevity anathema. Nathan Pritikin's substitute suggestion of 100 plus one's age is much better. In Japan, where the 1978 average life-span for males was 72.7 and that for females 77.9 years, the average cholesterol readings were three-fourths those considered normal by American standards. Cholesterol levels observed in Soviet Georgia and among populations with a low incidence of cardiovascular diseases show a consistent pattern of levels one-half to three-fourths of those thought normal in the developed world. Individuals who want to know their cholesterol levels should be aware that different laboratories use slightly different standards in their testing; so it is not possible to make automatic comparisons with published data; and it is best to stay with the same laboratory when keeping track of one's readings over a period of time.

With these considerations in mind, the decision whether to include dairy products in the diet becomes largely one of individual taste. As long as the entire fat content in the diet remains low, there is no observable harm in consuming some in the form of eggs, cream, or butter. Dairy products that have low fat content can be treated like any other food, and the case histories of longevous people show that many, including one Delina Filkins, used dairy products extensively throughout their long lives.

A predominantly vegetarian diet provides many automatic health bonuses. One of them is that the vitamin and mineral content will easily exceed the minimum daily requirements set by the Food and Drug Administration of the U.S. Public Health Service. Another is that raw foods, the basic component of vegetarian fare, cause minimal strain on the body, as they take only eighteen to twenty-four hours to go through the entire digestive process from ingestion to evacuation of any waste products. Cooked and processed foods need from eighty to one hundred hours to accomplish the same journey and may give off poisons while languishing for long periods in the lower intestinal tract. Development of constipation and hemorrhoids, chronic complaints of developed societies, is usually prevented or minimized by vegetarian diets because of the foods' high fiber content. Vegetarian foods produce large but soft stools that cleanse the tract and stimulate regular evacuation without strain.

An objection frequently raised to a vegetarian diet is that it provides insufficient protein. This view is based on at least two fallacies: that the body needs a large quantity of protein daily and that meat is its best source. There can be no question that protein is crucial to bodily well-being. Protein provides twenty-two essential amino acids, including eight which the body cannot synthesize. It is needed for growth, and it regulates the body's fluid balance. The minimum daily requirements for adults established by the Food and Agricultural Organization of the United Nations come to about 30 grams for the average adult female and 38 grams for adult males. The National Academy of Sciences in the United States recommends an additional 20 grams as a safety margin.

The American diet far exceeds these standards.[5] From 1900 to the end of the 1970s, with almost no change from year to year, the average American consumed between 88 and 104 grams of protein daily. Much of this came from meat, although protein is found in eggs, nuts, lentils, grains, brewer's yeast, beans, dairy products, seeds, and other foods. The danger of eating an otherwise nutritious and varied vegetarian diet and and not automatically receiving sufficient protein is nil.

The mystique of animal protein is nurtured by the fiction that it is needed to build muscle, an idea going back at least to ancient Greece, where Olympic athletes were taught to eat flesh if they wished to be champions. Contemporary football players and boxers, operating under the same conviction, often train on diets featuring steak two and three times a day. Yet the protein from vegetable sources provides the same acids as protein from meat, and the actual working of muscles to build new muscle requires energy that is best furnished by carbohydrates and fats. In terms of efficient use of available protein, eggs are 95 percent efficient, while beef, at 70 percent, barely noses out dried beans.

Vegetarian animals are the world's sturdiest creatures. The endurance of the camel, the strength of the ox, and the longevity of the tortoise are proverbial; and the bird with the longest life-span happens to be the parrot, a fruit and seed eater. In contests staged at the turn of the century in France and the United States, vegetarian athletes who were pitted against nonvegetarians came out ahead in most categories, including endurance and strength.[6] Numerous world and Olympic records are held by vegetarians, some in weight lifting. Barbara Moore undertook her walking feats partly to demonstrate the value of her vegetarian diet, and there are vegetarian athletes in all the major professional sports. Anyone still doubting the strength-building powers of vegetables might try to arm-wrestle a gorilla or put a flying tackle on an elephant.

If vegetable versus animal protein were a matter only of six of one versus half a dozen of the other, the choice could be left to individual taste; but there is mounting evidence that high protein consumption is another case in which more of a food is not only not better, but decidedly worse. Coaches have discovered that athletes who eat a protein-heavy diet and train vigorously are particularly subject to dehydration and heat stroke. This is so because high protein consumption increases the need for fluid—to wash out the by-products deposited when the protein is metabolized. A diet consistently high in protein puts a chronic burden on the kidneys and, to a lesser degree, the liver. High protein intake reduces the body's calcium and has been linked to various cancers and heart diseases.

Intensifying all of these danger factors is the adulteration of the animal products now sold in the marketplace. Any similarity between the modern cow, chicken, or turkey and those eaten in the nineteenth century is purely coincidental. Modern animals are forced to grow faster and fattier through chemicals. A notorious example of the hazards is the use of diethylstilbestrol (DES), which, although proved in 1947 to be carcinogenic, was injected directly into animals for another twenty-five years before being prohibited by federal mandate. DES is only one of fifteen sex hormones in use of which ten are proved or suspected carcinogens. Some, like DES and dienestrol diacetate, are so clearly linked to vaginal cancer that the Food and Drug Administration warns against their use. A number of scientists, not linked to the government, have speculated that the soaring rate of breast cancer in women may be related to the different hormones routinely pumped into animals slated for human consumption.

To this health concern may be added the dangers posed by scores of antibiotics and other drugs that are known to have a negative effect on the human organism. Some are injected directly into the animal, and others are added to feed. Virtually all turkey feed, 80 percent of feed used for swine, 80 percent of food given to calves, 60 percent of cattle feed, and 30 percent of chicken feed have these additives.[7] Still other additives, including sodium nitrate and sodium nitrite used to preserve and to color luncheon meats, are such firmly established carcinogens that several nations have followed the lead of Norway in banning their use. As the 1970s drew to an end, the U.S. Government reported that 14 percent of all meat and poultry had illegal residual levels of drugs and pesticides. Yet another hazard is posed by the seventy transmissible diseases carried by animals eaten by humans. The chance of infection is primarily guarded against by an antiquated and understaffed meat-inspection system which came into existence only after widespread abuses by meat-packers were publicized at the turn of the century.

Genetic alteration has overtaken the most commonly eaten animals. Cattle, probably more sacred in the United States than in India if for quite different reasons, have been reengineered to provide fat marbling throughout the body, giving beef its distinctive taste with no regard to the added burden on the human heart. That grand old American bird, the turkey, has been similarly altered, being reduced from six native breeds to one, a reshaped White Holland. The self-basting frozen creature widely sold at Thanksgiving and Christmas gets a significant portion of its weight from a cheap fattening injection of water and oil. More brutalized than either cattle or turkeys are chickens, most of which spend their entire lives in cages.

How meat is prepared, including "down home" favorites like fried chicken and barbecued ribs, creates more problems. Frying has already been identified as a peril to good digestion. Deep frying is worse. Barbecuing on a grill is somewhat easier on the system, but the portion of the meat coming into contact with the grill can become carcinogenic, as can all of the meat that becomes charred. People using chemically manufactured charcoal cubes instead of wood briquettes add more toxins, and the radiation hazards of the microwave ovens used to reheat or cook foods in many homes and commercial food outlets may be much greater than previously suspected. Unfortunately, few people can or want to connect their heavy meat consumption with premature aging or degenerative diseases.

Fish, crustaceans, and mollusks, generally, are treated as meat in terms of dietary components. Most crustaceans and mollusks are so high in cholesterol and fats that even with a rigorous daily work routine they must be regarded as treats. Fish have fewer inherent drawbacks if they can be found in uncontaminated waters; but this is increasingly difficult, as many streams and lakes and parts of the ocean have become polluted through chemical leaching and dumping. The most dangerous poisons in American waters are mercury and PCBs—polychlorinated biphenyls. Their threat is so immediate that much of the Great Lakes region has been closed to commerical fishing. Just examining a fish does not reveal whether it is contaminated. The buyer is left to trust in the fish seller's honesty, and more often than not the seller is without the means to certify the fish as safe for consumption.

The history of PCBs illustrates the magnitude of the toxic problem.[8] Since they were first made in 1930 by Monsanto for use as coolants and lubricants, 1.4 billion pounds of PCBs have been produced in the United States alone. Although questions about their harmful effect on the health of chemical workers were raised in the 1940s, it was not until the mid-1960s that PCBs that had slipped into the environment began to show up in the dead bodies of birds, fish, and animals. The warning alarm was first sounded in Sweden. Among the various problems traced to PCBs were bone deformities, cancer, and stillbirths. After the environmental movement made their production a political issue, the manufacture and sale of PCBs were banned under the terms of the Toxic Substance Control Act. Meanwhile, there were an estimated 150 million pounds remaining in the soil, water, and air, with another 290 million pounds in dumps and landfills. PCBs have been found in the Atlantic Ocean at depths below 10,000 feet.

In 1979, the same year the PCB ban went into effect, there was an accident at the Pierce Packing Company in Billings, Montana, which contaminated 1 million pounds of animal feed shipped to ranchers and farmers in nineteen states, some Canadian provinces, and Japan. At least 7 million eggs, 1 million chickens, 30,000 turkeys, 5,300 hogs,

2 million pounds of grease, and 74,000 bakery items had to be destroyed. The value of these products and the disposal and testing costs came to $10 million.[9] This catastrophic accident was similar to an incident in the Midwest a few years earlier that had severely contaminated dairy herds in Michigan. The culprit in that tragedy was polybrominated biphenyl or PBB, a fire retardant which got mixed into cattle feed.[10] Characteristically, the state department of agriculture's efforts in the matter amounted to a cover-up. It took a dairy farmer who also had a degree in chemistry to unravel the skein of guilt, eventually causing even Michigan's governor to recognize the problem and belatedly take action.

Chemical contamination of food reaches its zenith in the processed-and-packaged-food industries, where additives artificially flavor, color, and preserve foods. The overall purpose of these additives is to increase the product's profitability. The artificial flavor substitutes for expensive natural flavor; the artificial color cosmetically disguises what has happened to the food during processing; and the preservatives extend the product's shelf or warehouse life. How successfully the body can handle these additives is a matter of bitter dispute. But no one can dispute that few of the additives appeared in any food before 1930 or that they convey any discernible prolongevous benefit.

Additives acknowledged to be toxic or carcinogenic are common. Arguments bordering on criminal irresponsibility have been developed to the effect that the use of poisons in small quantities is harmless or an acceptable risk in view of the marketing advantages. However, different body chemistries have different tolerances for a poison, so when it comes to individual use, there can be no foolproof safety threshold. Furthermore, chemicals interact when combined, so that taking in several different sets of additives in different foods, even if they are safe in isolation, can have unpredictable and possibly adverse chemical consequences. Whether the additives hold down prices is questionable as well. Successful mass marketing existed before additives became widespread, and the most expensive foods on the market are exactly those prepackaged and processed products with the most additives and chemical alterations.

An individual with a good background in chemistry and lots of time might conceivably go through all the chemicals used in foods to determine which are safe, which are dubious, and which are definitely harmful. Among other tasks, this would require inquiries to each manufacturer to find out what general terms like stabilizers, emulsifiers, and artificial flavors (or colors) mean in specific chemical terms. Frequently, artificial substances are given clever names which obscure their nature. Hence, the artificial flavor "vanillin" is easily misread as the natural flavor "vanilla." Artificial products carry names like "Dairy Creme" or "Dairy Creamer" even though they are nondairy products.

The Food and Drug Administration is mandated to deal with adulterants in food, but it has been understaffed and underfunded for decades as well as being misunderstood by the public and harassed by the food industry. Despite the impression in the media that it is extremely difficult to get new additives onto the market, the FDA has a nearly impossible job trying to monitor the new chemicals constantly being proposed. In practice, rather than the manufacturer's having to prove or even guarantee the safety of additives, the FDA has to prove their possible ill effects. Despite these handicaps, the FDA has established a pattern in the use of additives that no person seeking long life dares ignore. Time and again, substances originally believed safe have proved to be extremely harmful. No fewer than fourteen of the sixteen approved food dyes of 1946 were banned as of 1980 on the ground that they were carcinogens. It seems clear that consumers are being asked to jeopardize their health in order to strengthen corporate balance sheets. One can only speculate on how much of the staggering annual medical bill might be attributable to "cost-saving" additives.

Processed foods are so low on the nutritional scoreboard to begin with that the risks posed by additives make them totally unacceptable. One can only hope that consumer rejection of such products will reach a high enough level to discourage producers from their use. The health-food boom has been something of a corrective to the trend in which more and more foods are tampered with; but terms like "natural" and "organic" need to be legally defined to prevent abuse. During the 1960s and '70s legislation spurred by health activists brought about better food labeling and strengthening of laws affecting product safety. Much more remains to be done, including the establishment of financial and even criminal liability on the part of manufacturers who suppress negative findings about the safety of what they sell as food. There are far too many excellent foods readily available for there to be any validity to the argument that some risks are acceptable or necessary. The plaint sometimes heard that any food eaten in sufficient quantities causes cancer is simply not true.

Fresh fruits and vegetables are not automatically safe either. Although DDT and other dangerous pesticides once widely used are now banned, there are still more than five thousand approved pesticides, waxes, and colorings. The safest way to avoid them, other than having a personal garden, is to patronize stores that sell only naturally grown products, which means the food was grown without benefit of chemicals or spraying—the way all food was grown previous to the twentieth century. While more expensive than regular produce, such natural foods, used exclusively in vegetarian meals, are cheaper than a typical meal with meat and processed food. A second option is to patronize a farmers' market. Small truck farmers usually employ more traditional methods, and it is possible to talk with them to discover what pesticides may have been used. Very rarely will they wax or color their products. Untreated dried fruits and nuts are available in most areas, but one has to examine the packages carefully or ask questions about the use of preservatives. Simply shopping at a health-food store or selecting packaging with health-food appeals on it is no guarantee of safety. Many profit-oriented concerns have tried to take advantage of the high prices commanded by quality food without providing the kind of purity desired.

Fortunately, most pesticides, as claimed, do not penetrate the skin of plants, so thorough washing adds a considerable margin of safety. Even when a shopper is thrown back on produce grown by agribusiness, the danger of consuming toxins is much less than with processed foods and meats. The least chemical contamination occurs at the lower end of the food chain. Thus root vegetables and grains have only fractional retention of pollutants, but meat, fish, and poultry, all found at the opposite end, can be high. Legumes, fruits, and vegetables of all kinds also have relatively low retention. Dairy products are midway between the various meat and nonmeat categories.

A predominantly vegetarian diet will not necessarily be a low-fat diet. If one is consuming dairy products or large quantities of nuts, there is ample opportunity to ice cream, cashew, and butter oneself into a cardiac condition. Among the major problems associated with excessive fat intake are tendencies to atherosclerosis, gout, obesity, and diabetes, as well as the various illnesses connected with high levels of cholesterol, triglycerides, and uric acid. High-fat diets have been linked to cancer of the breast and colon, but it is not clear how much of the danger is due to the fat itself and how much to additives that may have found their way into the fat. To protect against these hazards, within the schema of lowered overall caloric intake, no more than 15 percent should come from fat, which has about 9 calories per gram. This 15-percent target is half of what has been called for by government experts, but such authorities tend to set goals that do not appear too severe to the fat-gobbling American public. Saturated fats, in particular, should be avoided whenever possible.

Americans also can't seem to get enough sugar, consuming about 2 pounds a week, one-fourth directly and three-fourths as part of processed foods. The excess pounds burdening many bodies are caused by this sugar overload. Some degenerative diseases and the hyperactive behavior of many children have been traced to a high sugar intake. Perhaps the most insidious effect of sugar is that it debases the palate. When there is no strong addiction to sugar, what tastes good is usually nutritious, but as one develops a sugar habit, only what tastes sweet is thought to taste good. Overweight but undernourished sugar junkies are not uncommon. A typical daily routine for many Americans begins with a sugar hit at breakfast. This overstimulates the pancreas, sending out large quantities of insulin which set up reactions that lead to the midmorning feeling of depression which is then interpreted as the need for more sugar. Cutting down or eliminating sugar from breakfast disrupts the self-perpetuating sugar cycle at its source. In pursuing this objective, one has to be wary of the various names manufacturers use for sugar. Sucrose, corn sweetener, fructose, dextrose, and sorbital are all sugars.

The sugar found in natural food is sufficient for bodily functions, so it is unnecessary to use additional sugar except as a taste supplement. The wholly refined white sugar found in most homes is the most difficult sugar for the body to handle and should be avoided. Partly refined brown sugar, the staple of many health-conscious households, is not much better. Honey or molasses, both of which contain minerals and vitamins, pose fewer digestive difficulties, but should never be thought of as health foods, and their use should be held to a minimum. The most easily handled and most useful sugars are those which are found in fruit. An apple or orange in the morning will give one a better start than a sugar-coated bakery product. Sugar taken as fruit has the advantage of coming in a bulky form which makes excessive consumption less likely.

The artificial sweeteners, cyclamates and saccharin, place one in double jeopardy. Independent scientific organizations have shown both to be carcinogenic, and both keep alive the acquired taste for sweets. One of the ironies of saccharin consumption is that because of the way saccharin chemically reacts with fat cells, it may increase the desire to eat in overweight people. Saccharin's use by heavy smokers is especially dangerous because of a synergistic reaction which intensifies the harmful effects of tobacco.

Salt, formerly used mainly as a preservative, shares many of the characteristics of sugar as a palate debaser. Its use to satisfy an acquired taste may lead to horrendous nutritional choices. Some recipes that now feature large quantities of sugar and salt can be traced historically through cookbooks to precursor recipes requiring neither flavoring in any significant amount, if at all. Although it is not understood how sodium influences blood pressure, studies of more than twenty cultures show there was no hypertension where there was limited salt consumption. This and other evidence has led physicians to caution high-blood-pressure patients, among others, to reduce their salt intake or eliminate salt from their diet altogether. For the would-be longevous, salt, like sugar, should rarely be added to food.

Processed foods are sodium holocausts which the 34 million Americans with high blood pressure should be particularly concerned about. When Consumers Union examined common products not normally thought of as salty, it made some surprising discoveries: a 1-ounce serving of Kellogg's Corn Flakes was found to contain twice as much sodium as an ounce of Planter's Cocktail Peanuts; two slices of Pepperidge Farm White Bread contained more sodium than a 1-ounce bag of Lay's Potato Chips; and one-half cup of Jell-O Chocolate Flavor Instant Pudding had more sodium than three slices of Oscar Mayer Bacon. Other packaged foods high in salt included tuna fish, tomato sauce, beans and franks, cottage cheese, salad dressing, hamburgers, pickles, tomato juice, and sweet peas.[11]

A final category of solid foods worthy of specific comment is that of natural ones considered to have medicinal powers. Examples would include curry, paprika, various peppers, horseradish, onions, and garlic. Some of these are natural antibiotics, but they all tend to jolt the body by irritating one membrane or another. Often they cause tearing, sneezing, or a burning sensation in the stomach. Contrary to popular mythology, there is no bodily accommodation to this process. In fact, some taste buds are destroyed, necessitating greater quantities of the irritant to produce the original taste effect. Districts of India and Mexico where highly seasoned food is preferred have a high incidence of stomach ailments. Some vegetarians argue that spicy foods in moderation have a place in the diet, but most maintain that the jolt would not be required by a properly functioning organism. There is no conclusive research on the possible negative or positive longevity impact of such foods, so using them is a matter of taste preference. But if an individual's metabolism reacts unfavorably, their use should be discontinued immediately.

Liquids should be judged by the same criteria applied to solid foods. Healthful drinks include unadulterated fruit juices, vegetable juices, mineral water, milk (skim or buttermilk preferred), and plain water. The body's appestat will indicate the desirable quantities unless there is artificial stimulation from salt or sweeteners. Soda pop is to be avoided because of its many chemical additives, colas being the worst because of their high caffeine and sugar content. A twist of lime or a dash of freshly squeezed lemon juice in naturally carbonated mineral water provides a thirst quencher whose only additives are a trace of vitamins and minerals.

A peculiar situation pertains to alcohol. Heavy consumption seriously damages various parts of the body, particularly the brain and the liver, and alcohol in any quantity accelerates the body's ability to assimilate fat. Alcohol also interacts with cigarette fumes in a way that increases the carcinogenic effect of smoking. In spite of these negative effects of either heavy consumption of alcohol or consumption in combination with smoking, moderate drinkers who do not smoke are less likely to suffer heart attacks than abstainers or heavy drinkers.[12] Consumption of alcohol is relatively common among centenarians: one may recall the jigger of applejack taken every morning in Abkhasia, the daily half-pint of potato brew enjoyed by Shigechiyo Izumi, the wines consumed by Luigi Cornaro, and the occasional brandy favored by the ladies of Cambridgeshire.

The benefits of alcohol, especially for older people, are linked to its ability to arouse the appetite, to stimulate the heart, and to expand the arterial walls. One study of wine drinking in eighteen developed nations concluded that protection for the heart might be linked to some constituent of the wine other than alcohol, but most researchers believe the benefits are at least partly due to an increase alcohol causes in the number of alpha lipids. Although news reporters like to write stories of hard-drinking old-timers, it must be emphasized that the advantages of drinking are not so grand that a taste for alcohol should be deliberately cultivated. But if alcohol is part of the diet, moderate consumption may have some prolongevous benefits. "Moderate" may be about nine shots of distilled spirits, a dozen cans of beer, or fourteen glasses of wine a week. Higher consumption should be avoided; and it is advisable to have some food when drinking.

Mixed drinks are a poor way of taking alcohol, because of the sugar and additives employed to give them distinctive flavors. Traditional beer made with heavy malt tended to be rich in Vitamin E, but modern brewing methods have pretty much denutritionalized the drink. In addition, beer and Scotch whisky have been found to contain nitrosamines, a family of potent carcinogens. In any case, heavy beer drinking is inadvisable, as the excessive water intake involved stresses the kidneys and other organs.

The modern passion for caffeine is another example of a new fuel that does not necessarily constitute progress. Among the numerous effects of caffeine are a depletion of the B vitamins and irritation of the urinary and anal tracts. The major source for adults, of course, is coffee, but caffeine also appears in cocoa, chocolate, cola drinks, and some teas. A small glass of cola has about half the amount of caffeine there is in a cup of coffee, and a chocolate bar about a fourth. This means that when overall body size is considered, a child drinking two glasses of cola a day and eating two chocolate bars has a caffeine intake equivalent to eight cups of coffee for an adult. Taking caffeine as a means of "settling down" is biological nonsense, for one of its chief effects is to irritate the nervous system and stomach. Even the drinking of caffeine to stay awake while driving is somewhat self-defeating, as the body will suffer depression about an hour after taking in the caffeine, calling for a new hit.

Drinking tea is not necessarily a good alternative. Many teas, particularly those thought of as brisk, contain nearly as much caffeine as coffee does. Tea also may contain catechin tannin, which has been shown to cause oral and esophageal cancer. This danger is avoided if the tea is taken with milk, which binds the tannin. Herbal mixtures are not the health miracles often advertised either. A few contain carcinogens, and many that yield medicinal benefits do so because of an unusual concentration of acids. Using such brews on a regular basis is like taking penicillin daily. Anyone determined to use tea as a regular drink needs to study the particular leaves involved. Most Chinese teas, for example, do not contain tannin; most Indian teas do.

While caffeine has no positive input in the diet, its consumption in very moderate quantities may not be particularly deleterious. As long as a person can limit caffeine intake from all sources to the equivalent of two cups of coffee a day, it is far more important to concentrate on reducing the intake of fats, sugars, sodium, and artificial additives. This emphasis is particularly advisable for persons who find it psychologically difficult to eliminate coffee in one stage. Decaffeinated coffee also could be used for psychological support, but since the harmful effects of coffee are not limited to its caffeine content, decaffeinated coffee is not a good long-term solution. As the body becomes chemically tuned to an upgraded diet, coffee will usually cause headaches, consciousness of the heartbeat, stomach upsets, and other unpleasant reactions which will facilitate its final termination as a habitual item of consumption.

Some health manuals advocate that the variety of food in the total diet be limited, with only a few foods eaten at any given meal. Although this idea has a poetic appeal because of its simplicity, a monodiet does not make nutritional sense. Primitive peoples ate a much wider range of plants and fruits than people in modern societies do, and the diversity of foods the stomach can accommodate with ease suggests that variety was genetically intended. Singling out a narrow band of food to be the fuel of the body runs the risk of excluding an adequate amount of known and unknown essential nutrients. Other than the common-sense avoidance of combining foods that produce volatile chemical reactions, there are no particular advantages to eating only one or two foods per sitting.

How often one should eat is a more pertinent concern. The nibbling pattern would seem to be the most natural, as that is the way most animals in nature eat, but there is no evidence that a limited number of formal meals is harmful. The three-major-meals-a-day pattern, which is based on the economic organization of modern society, is acceptable. Far more relevant is that the largest caloric intake occur early in the working day. Borrowing an often-used group of similes, it is best to breakfast like a lion, lunch like a squirrel, and dine like a bird. The rationale is that food not burned for energy will be stored as fat or excreted. The more calories taken late in the day, the more the body is forced to work needlessly. Although many psychological dependencies have been built around late eating or midnight snacks, the physical consequences can be extremely negative. The would-be longevous should fuel up early, use the fuel during the course of the day, and go to sleep without forcing new internal housekeeping chores on the tired body.

Another need allied with regular eating habits is evacuation, the subject of more jokes than almost any other bodily function. While great individual variations are possible, even

light eaters should expect one bowel movement each day.
However, only when one feels bloated or uncomfortable
should less frequency be a matter of concern. In that case,
within the context of highly regularized eating times, there
should be an increase in raw foods in the diet, an increase in
foods with high fiber content, and an increase in liquids.
Exercises that put pressure on the lower abdomen also can be
employed, as long as one follows the usual exercise precautions. Should these responses fail to achieve regularity, then
it is much wiser to consult a physician to see what may be
the trouble than to get into the laxative habit, which has
long-term negative effects.

The pivotal prolongevous meal is breakfast, for it is at
breakfast that the day's eating cycle is established. What is
considered a proper breakfast food is just a matter of con-
vention, a doughnut and coffee hardly being more natural
than a plate of vegetables or a fruit salad and soup. As a
prelude to a vigorous day in distant fields, many traditional
farming families used to have mammoth breakfasts comparable to modern dinners. Lumberjacks packing away piles of
pancakes before going into the woods were meeting similar
needs. Complex carbohydrates such as cereal and breads that
will release energy throughout the day at a regular pace are
superior to the illusionary lift of sugar and coffee hits. Fruits,
nuts, and preserves can be included for immediate energy, but
any food that is prolongevously rational is fine. To be avoided
in most cases is an extremely light breakfast, which tends to
set up a delayed-eating cycle culminating in a late dinner.

The temperature and speed at which foods are consumed
are secondary factors in terms of extending life, yet worthy of
some consideration. A fast meal is nearly always a poor meal.
Everyone has had the inside of his or her mouth burned by
something eaten too hot, or has experienced a headache from
eating something too cold. These extremes are bodily hints
that, by and large, food and drink are best consumed at the
temperatures most commonly found in nature. This does not
preclude hot drinks, frozen desserts, soups, or chilled fruits,

but it does suggest that they be held to a minimum. Slowing down does more than prevent burned mouths and headaches. Digestion commences in the mouth, with chewing and salivation. If this process is bypassed by bolting food or washing it down with liquids, more work is required later in the system by parts of the body less suited to the task. Fast eating also can outpace the stomach's ability to signal the brain that enough fuel has been ingested—one reason second helpings often feel less satisfying. Once again, the folk customs of Abkhasia are pertinent; the Abkhasians believe it is impolite to eat rapidly or to eat large portions.

Taken item by item, few of the dietary changes indicated by longevous considerations are extreme or difficult. As a totality, however, the diet is quite distinct. Unlike faddish plans which promote rapid weight loss by temporarily upsetting the normal chemical relationships within the body, the prolongevous diet aims to provide the variety, quality, and quantity of fuels that will sustain the most efficient and beneficial reactions. The systematic reduction of fats, salt, sugars, and additives will produce innumerable chemical adjustments within the body. Gradual weight loss will be the most visible side effect. Rushing these changes along would be a grave error. In addition to the organism's dislike of abrupt changes, because of the internal chaos they entail, there are many psychological and social pressures to contend with.

The shift to a prolongevous eating pattern begins with the reduction or elimination of the highest-risk items. While these are being dealt with on a priority basis, other poor but less destructive ones can continue. A period of more than a year may be needed to work through all the major required changes, with the speed dictated by individual personality and the quality of the starting diet. Time will be needed for friends and acquaintances to accept new habits. Among the most difficult persons to deal with may be close relatives or parents who insist that their brand of home cooking, however meat-and-fat oriented, is essential to good health and who feel insulted if it is declined. A somewhat cowardly but effective approach to maintaining a prolongevous diet without giving offense is to say that one is under a physician's orders. Another may be to eat strictly vegetarian meals at home, but to be more flexible in business or social settings.

The major reference needed to shape a diet is a manual that lists the caloric and nutritional values of the most common foods. After a few weeks this guide need not be consulted very often, but as even among the best-informed there are many misconceptions about food, it is prudent to look up any food frequently eaten rather than proceed on assumptions. Checking on specific foods is indicated also when there is a problem with weight control or insufficient energy. The following twelve points can serve as a dietary guideline:

1. Set a caloric intake that will maintain body weight at the desired prolongevous level or that will move one's weight toward that level at the rate of no less than a quarter-pound and no more than a full pound a week. For most persons this will be accomplished on a diet ranging between 1,500 and 2,500 calories daily. The caloric intake, however, will be greatly influenced by the amount of daily physical exertion.
2. Work toward a dietary balance of 10–15 percent fat, 10–15 percent protein, and 70–80 percent carbohydrates.
3. Emphasize high-quality foods, such as fresh vegetables, fresh fruit, and whole grains.
4. Hold meat, fish, or poultry consumption to once or twice a week. They are best served in combination with vegetables, as in a stew, or as a kind of garnish, as in Oriental cooking.
5. Eat raw foods whenever possible. Otherwise, the food may be steamed, boiled, or baked. Avoid frying.
6. Avoid all preservatives, artificial flavorings, artificial colorings, and other food additives.

7. Take in the largest amount of calories early in the workday. Keep all late eating to a minimum, and never eat just before going to sleep. Try to regularize mealtimes.

8. Hold salt consumption to a minimum. Be aware that salt can be a significant ingredient in many prepared foods.

9. Hold sugar consumption to a minimum. Be aware that sugar often slips into the diet under different names.

10. Drink only moderate amounts of alcohol.

11. Avoid caffeine.

12. Eat slowly.

The achievement of a prolongevous diet is a long-term process and not a single revolutionary act of the will. At any given point, it is sufficient to be replacing some nutritionally negative items with more positive ones. An unavoidable period of trial and error is necessary to find new food combinations, eating habits, beverages, and other dietary components that are truly satisfying, for it is essential that the new diet be enjoyable. If the diet is viewed as a sacrifice of good living, then it is not likely to be maintained. Indulgences like ice cream and pastry do not have to be altogether eliminated, and reducing their frequency to satisfy caloric and fat guidelines is immensely facilitated by the gradualist approach. The process has one built-in advantage in that as the diet becomes nutritionally superior, there is a corresponding surge in general health and a tendency for the body to react poorly to improper fuels. Perhaps there will never be a time when eating habits and knowledge of what is best reach 100-percent consistency, but with conscious effort, most people can come close. The more the real diet and the ideal diet come into confluence, the better the longevity prospects.

10

BIOCHEMICAL INDIVIDUALITY

> The sensitivity of various people to our *artificial* drugs seems to be fairly uniform. Not so the sensitivity to vitamins. There seem to be people who are unable to absorb or store them, and such people may develop symptoms of a vitamin deficiency on a diet which is completely satisfactory to others.
>
> —*Albert Szent-Györgyi*

The biochemical individuality of each human being is as distinct as a fingerprint. Differences in the basal metabolic rate are only the most obvious expression of particularism. For example, two-thirds of all humans have three arteries branching from the aorta, while the remaining third may have one, two, four, five, or even six. Similarly, the weight of the liver in relation to the rest of the body varies by sevenfold. Such differences in structure and mass are found in virtually all organs and systems of the body and greatly influence specific nutritional needs for any given person.[1]

Nutritional needs are further affected by a myriad of other factors. Illnesses almost always require at least a temporary increase in essential nutrients, because of the damage done both by the disease and by the drugs used to treat it. Pregnant women, older persons, and those living in areas with poor soil may require additional mineral intakes, while urban dwellers coping with foul air and potent virus strains may require extra vitamin protection. Awareness of realities of this kind has led many to add supplements and medications to their diets. However, the process of selection is often foolhardy.

Instead of consulting professional sources, most people put their trust in popular health books or articles in health magazines. Although such literature can provide a useful theoretical orientation to nutrition as well as a grasp of the nutritive value of specific foods, it cannot be relied on for making serious decisions about health. The major problem is that the data offered are usually contained in breezy simplifications of experimental research. The tentative nature of the conclusions, or the narrowness of the sample base in the original research, is often overlooked. The secondary author also rarely stresses the unknown long-term effects of increased use of a vitamin or mineral or fails to emphasize that, as with alcohol, what is sometimes beneficial in small doses may be quite harmful in larger ones. Nor do such authors appreciate the risk that increased intake of one vitamin or mineral often necessitates increased intake of others. The better health writers, who do try to account for this phenomenon, often propose a supplementary balancing act that leaves most people dizzy and is much too finely tuned for the present state of medical knowledge.

Recommendations on supplements tend to run in faddish cycles. Claims get rephrased with increasingly enthusiastic language in much the way the Hunza myth was propagated. The result is that some substances become widely used before basic research on them is conclusive. In the 1970s selenium was optimistically heralded as a possible cancer preventive because of some preliminary research and statistical data relating low rates of cancer to cultures with a relatively high intake of the mineral. Then other research indicated that selenium in large doses might cause cancer, could damage the central nervous system, and probably fostered dental problems. The continued uncertainty about selenium is not unique. Because some supplements are discussed widely and sold over the counter, consumers have been lulled into using them, regarding their safety with a suspension of disbelief they would never grant to the synthetic chemicals found in processed foods.

The starting point for judging the need for any vitamin or mineral supplement is the minimum daily requirement set by the health agencies of the federal government. Below these requirement levels, a specific disease of malnutrition will develop in almost all persons. Meeting the minimum daily requirement, however, does not necessarily rule out the possibility that higher amounts will be advisable, or that specific body chemistries or living situations warrant spectacular variations. A paradigm for judging whether to add a vitamin or mineral supplement to the diet can be established by considering the most widely supplemented nutrients: Vitamin E, Vitamin C, iron, and calcium.

Vitamin E has been extolled as a youth-giving substance because of its role as an antioxidant. By keeping cellular garbage from clogging the bloodstream, E promotes healthier skin tissue and better circulation. Less visible is its activity against free radicals, atoms that have broken off from other molecules and career through the system like cue balls on a billiard table. They split other molecules, creating more free radicals and disrupting orderly cellular life. Vitamin E halts this destruction by binding free radicals. It works in a similar fashion against substances like lead and ozone breathed into the body as constituents of polluted air.

Soviet gerontologists have long used E in their experimental diets and programs. Unlike BHA and BHT, synthetic antioxidants used in packaging materials, or the natural mineral selenium, even in high doses E has no observable negative effects. Among the best natural sources for the vitamin are whole grains and green leafy vegetables. One health writer has remarked that a rather poor Londoner of the nineteenth century who drank a few pints of malt beer and ate brown bread took in far more E than his or her contemporary counterpart. Yet it is precisely in the polluted modern metropolis that the need for E is greatest. This appears to be one situation in which an unnatural environmental condition may call for an unnatural quantity of a vitamin as a countermeasure. Determining the minimum daily requirement for E is difficult, as no particular disease seems to result from its absence. Until research is more conclusive, increase in the consumption of E should be mainly in the choice of natural foods, with a possible intake of from 100 to 400 international units daily as a supplement in environments where air quality is poor or there are high levels of background radiation.

Even more controversial than the use of E is the resort to tablets of ascorbic acid, or, as it is more commonly called, Vitamin C. The minimum daily requirement set by the U.S. government is 60 milligrams for adults, the level below which the disease of scurvy occurs; but the best-known booster of Vitamin C, Dr. Linus Pauling, Nobel Laureate in Chemistry for 1954, has written that the level most adults should be taking is between 2 and 4 grams![2] A difference of this magnitude among professional scientists is startling, to say the least. Almost as startling are the claims advanced in behalf of the vitamin. Ascorbic acid is said to prevent colds, to combat the harmful effects of carbon monoxide, to improve circulation, to aid in the healing of wounds, and to promote health in various organs. In addition, it has an undeniable synergistic effect when combined with E, making that vitamin far more potent than when it is taken alone.

Pauling believes that getting proper amounts of C into the diet would add from four to six years to the average lifespan—two to three from the prevention of the damage done by colds and another two to three from the improvement in general health. These gains would result from the use of ascorbic acid as a food supplement, a role that must be differentiated from its possible utilization as a medicine. One of the justifications offered by Pauling for his recommendations is based on a diet we have already identified as prolongevous. Pauling has calculated that on a diet of 2,500 calories coming only from fresh natural plant food, 2.3 grams of C would be available. Such a diet, of course, is not possible for most people in contemporary society, as vitamins are destroyed by modern methods of picking, marketing, and processing. Picking crops while they are green so that they can ripen on the way to market and the long delay between field and table greatly reduces their C content. Processing wipes out most of the vitamin in prepared foods, as does cooking at high temperatures, particularly in the presence of certain trace metals.

The optimal dose of C also is subject to the kind of biochemical individuality that affects all nutrients. Pauling thinks that a few people may get on quite well with as little as 250 milligrams daily, while others may require as much as 10 grams. He emphasizes that all available evidence shows C to be one of the least toxic substances consumed by humans. Although minor side effects sometimes occur when mega-doses are taken, there has never been a case of serious illness or death resulting from eating too much of it. Intriguing speculations have been advanced as to why the human body cannot manufacture its own C and whether C is properly classified as a vitamin. But the worst consequence of oversupplying C would seem to be that it is passed out through the urine without being used.[3]

Some scientists have hypothesized that C may be a kind of general or universal antitoxin which rallies bodily defense mechanisms. Soviet experts have been using it in combination with E in their longevity programs, and work is under way in various nations to see if ascorbic acid has a role to play in the treatment of gallstones, arthritis, diabetes, atherosclerosis, senility, and other ailments. In several countries, massive doses of C have been used to treat terminally ill cancer patients. The results have been more positive than those for more conventional therapies.[4] In relation to cold prevention the findings are indeterminate, but advocates claim that an intake of about 3 grams a day will prevent colds in most people. They note that even if far more of the vitamin is consumed than is needed, the danger is infinitesimal compared with the dangers known to accompany continued use of nonprescription cold fighters such as analgesics and antihistamines. Compared with C, aspirin, one of the most widely used drugs, is quite sinister. Regular use of aspirin will lead to internal bleeding, and in doses of 20 to 30 grams it is lethal.

Without necessarily accepting the most optimistic views of the qualities of C, it makes longevous sense to put large amounts of it into the diet, either through choice of foods or in combination with a supplement. Bodily reactions should be the prime method of determining how much is taken, with the 2.3 grams suggested by the raw diet a better starting point than the amount needed to prevent scurvy. Any factors that may deplete intake of the vitamin or increase its need would suggest temporary increases in the supplement. Most certainly, ascorbic acid should be the preferred method of dealing with colds and headaches and should be used as an auxiliary defense, because of its synergistic effect against any of the environmental toxins that call for the use of E. Foods rich in C can be found in any nutritional chart, but some with the highest concentration are broccoli spears, black currants, kale, parsley, and peppers.

Minerals are inorganic substances of a quite different nature from vitamins. Although some of them, usually in extremely small amounts, are essential to bodily functions, in higher quantities most minerals become harmful and will cause depletion of other nutrients. A diet featuring plant foods and some dairy products will easily satisfy all the known mineral requirements of the body. Nonetheless, the pressures of advertising and health gossip have made mineral supplements a highly profitable industry.

Probably the most commonly supplemented mineral is iron. The syndrome of "tired blood" and the higher iron needs of women and children have been widely publicized. Any real iron deficiency, however, is largely the result of the high percentage of refined foods in the typical modern diet. If more iron is needed, far better than any supplement would be an increase in the intake of natural foods rich in the mineral. Should that tactic fail to produce the desired results, the problem is likely to be not the amount of iron available for use but the body's inability to use it—a matter for a doctor, not an over-the-counter salesperson, to deal with.

Calcium, the most prevalent mineral in the body and the main component of bones, is another widely supplemented mineral. Yet there is little chance of calcium deficiency in people who use dairy products. If those foods are restricted for any reason, a conscious effort should be made to ensure that the required daily intake of 800 milligrams is being met. This is far from difficult. Three ounces of sardines (with bones) provide 372 milligrams, and a cup of shelled almonds provides 332. Servings of dandelion, mustard, turnip, or collard greens are nearly as good. Any comprehensive nutritional chart will yield combinations of calcium-bearing foods that will negate the need for supplements such as bone meal or dolomite.

Calcium deficiencies quite often are only tangentially problems of supply. High intakes of fat hinder the body's ability to absorb calcium, while high intakes of animal protein result in excessive calcium losses through urination. More fundamentally, Vitamin D must be present in the body for calcium to be absorbed through the intestinal wall, so those who are low in that vitamin for any reason must make appropriate adjustments. Also, when large amounts of other minerals, such as the phosphorus used in baby formulas, are ingested, the need for calcium will increase accordingly.

Whenever the immediate bodily needs for calcium fall below the daily supply, the body will borrow the mineral from the bones and the teeth. A chronic deficiency will produce deformed bones in children and soft bones in adults. Conversely, although a moderate oversupply of calcium can be usefully stored in the bones, continued overdoses create health problems of their own. The rule to follow with calcium and all other mineral supplements is to avoid them unless their use is prescribed and monitored by a physician.

Seeking medical advice on supplements opens the whole question of the role the practicing physician should play in the longevity project. The ideal professional would regard the physician–patient dynamic as a partnership. The emphasis would be on the maintenance of health rather than on the prevention or cure of disease. One historical precedent for this kind of relationship can be found in ancient China, where a healer was paid only as long as the patient remained in good health. Unfortunately, today's focus is on treating disease. Medical schools place such a strong emphasis on surgical procedures and powerful drugs that they all but ignore nutrition and other means that might allow the body to maintain good health with its own resources. Once a doctor goes into practice, pharmaceutical and medical-equipment firms continue the orientation begun in medical school. The system is further reinforced by patients who put off seeking assistance until they are obviously ill, patients who want quick cures, and patients who are lacking in personal discipline, like high-blood-pressure victims who won't lose weight or heart-disease and emphysema victims who won't stop smoking.

The search to find the right physician requires more effort than allowing one's fingers to meander through the professional pages of the telephone directory or than accepting the services of those who have treated friends or family. Even a physician known to have a nutritional perspective may simply prescribe supplements with the same abandon with which other physicians dispense penicillin or Valium. The more realistic approach to securing good medical advice is to find a traditional but sensitive physician who can be made to feel that the would-be longevous individual offers a positive change of pace from everyday routines and an opportunity to observe the long-term effects of naturalistic health practices. Such a physician should be prepared to answer many questions and to have long consultations with the patient.

One of the first services many would-be longevous people will require is a determination of whether any organic problems prevent them from undertaking the longevity agenda, particularly the exercise component. When going over test findings, it is not acceptable to be informed that the results are normal. Exact numbers should be obtained, and they should be related to longevous, not conventional, standards. During and after the transformation to a prolongevous profile, some people will feel more comfortable if changes going on in the body are monitored periodically. A suitable checklist and timetable can be worked out with the physician. The patient should make it clear that he or she is willing to pay for the time and expertise involved, just as someone else may be paying for surgery, medication, or bedside consultations.

Prolongevous ground rules should be established firmly during the initial diagnostic period. For example, the annual checkup advised by many health professionals can be a physical ordeal. Doctors working with older patients have questioned the desirability of many of the procedures involved, because they greatly fatigue or discomfort their patients. Such doubts should be extended across the entire age spectrum. Especially dubious are tests that result in a painful reaction, although that is not the sole criterion.

That a test is standard procedure is no guarantee of safety. The diagnostic X-rays routinely ordered by doctors, dentists, and chiropractors provide a chilling example. Using language designed to make science accessible to the average person, Dr. Priscilla Laws has written an analysis of the dangers posed by X-rays.[5] She has shown that diagnostic X-rays currently constitute the largest source of humanly created radiation exposure and that a person who receives a complete series of abdominal X-rays may easily exceed the annual occupational safety limit. Moreover, what is considered a safe dosage has been revised spectacularly downward for more than eighty years. In the 1910s and 1920s, 10 rems a day was considered an acceptable exposure. By 1936 an advisory committee had lowered the rate to 30 rems a *year*. In 1957 the National Committee on Radiation Protection and Measurement lowered the acceptable amount to 5 rems a year. Alarmed by the steady rise in background radiation and the increasing incidence of cancer, many public-health activists believe the present standards are still too generous.

In the introduction to Law's study, Dr. Sidney M. Wolfe of the Health Research Group summarized the alarming conclusions in studies on radiation safety made by the Department of Health, Education and Welfare. These reports found that 20 percent of all X-ray units inspected were not in compliance with state laws, the result being that patients were exposed to excessive and illegal amounts of radiation. Over 90 percent of all medical X-rays were being given without proper shielding, and about 50 percent overexposed the patients because the beam was much larger than needed. Dentists who had completed their professional training prior to 1940 were found to be exposing their patients to twice as much radiation as dentists who graduated after 1965. A subsequent study completed by the Food and Drug Administration's Bureau of Radiation Health in 1979 was just as disturbing. The survey, which covered forty-five states, showed that of 35,224 dental X-ray units inspected, 36 percent used exposures that were "excessively high," and even among the 3,152 new units inspected, 61 percent were not in compliance with federal regulations.[6]

So many other medical practices have hazards associated with them that the term "iatrogenic disease" has been coined to indicate a mental or physical disorder caused by medical personnel. Some of the major contemporary iatrogenic reactions stem from ineffective vaccines, laboratory errors, faulty diagnostic devices, overdoses of medication, and useless treatments. Medical schools are concerned with the phenomenon, but it is as old as the profession and as predictable as human fallibility. Even under the best of circumstances, favored techniques often include deliberately inflicting pain, poisoning the body, or taking other calculated risks.

Considering the stakes involved, before agreeing to any medical intervention the patient who is oriented to long life must insist on detailed information on how that intervention affects the body, any known risks, and viable alternatives. Any procedure which involves a serious invasion of the body is particularly suspect. If faced with a disturbing diagnosis or proposed course of treatment, the patient should seek a second or third opinion before making a final decision. Although chemical or surgical remedies may not be avoidable, if reasonable options are available they should be seriously considered, whatever the apparent inconvenience.

The methods used to treat high blood pressure in the past forty years provide an insight into how the newest and easiest treatment isn't always the best treatment. During the 1940s it was established that sodium intake had an adverse effect on hypertension. Restricted-sodium diets became the treatment of the day. In 1957 various medicines that acted directly on the nerves and blood vessels without requiring sodium restriction were developed and quickly became the favored treatment. By the 1970s the new drugs were found to be creating negative side effects, and many physicians returned to the sodium-restriction approach, especially when the medication would have to be taken for a substantial period of time. Of further concern was the growing tendency to treat mild or borderline cases of hypertension with drugs, subjecting the patients to needless risk.

Another example of the dangers of introducing drugs into the body on a regular basis is found in the use of estrogen in birth-control pills and as a treatment for menopausal distress and other disorders. Although this particular hormone has been used in longevity work in the Soviet Union and can have an immediate "rejuvenating" effect, long-term use increases the risks of developing cancer and heart disease. The use of synthetic hormones by pregnant women in the

1940s and '50s produced birth defects. In view of this record, prolonged use of hormones is unwise. Women using birth-control pills should switch to other methods if possible, especially if use continues for more than two years. At a minimum, women should be certain they are getting a birth-control formula with the least amount of estrogen necessary.

In addition to direct negative effects on the body, medication may also deplete the organism of minerals and vitamins. The digitalis used by many heart patients affects potassium and thiamine needs. Diuretics affect Vitamin B, Vitamin C, calcium, magnesium, potassium, and zinc requirements. Mineral oil and commonly used drugs like aspirin, barbiturates, antacids, and antibiotics cause nutritional depletions. Occasional use of such substances is hardly cause for alarm, but if they are used habitually, mineral and vitamin supplements of some kind may be in order. The negative effects of many drugs were first observed in older patients who had used them for a considerable time or whose restricted diets or failing health made them susceptible to deficiencies.

In short, no supplement or medication should ever be taken until there is a demonstrated need established by bodily symptoms which have been judged against professional medical literature or by consultations with a physician. The exceptions to this are situations in which the need has been demonstrated before any symptoms can develop. For example, because iodine deficiency in the soil is known to encourage goiter, it would be foolish for persons in such geographic situations to wait for signs of the disease before adding some iodine to their diet. The possible use of C and E supplements is linked to similar evaluations of the quality of the food supply and the hostile nature of the industrial environment. At some future time, when nutritional science is more fully developed, it will be possible to pinpoint prolongevous nutritional elements and adjust the diet accordingly. Even then, and most certainly until then, it is best to get vitamins and minerals from natural foods, in which the combination of nutrients, their form, and as yet unknown factors are more likely to be positive than in commercial pills produced for profit. If, as the evidence strongly suggests, restricted caloric intake adds to long life, a rule of thumb for identifying how much of any given nutrient is needed would be to determine how much of it would be available in a 2,500-caloric diet made up of raw foods. Unless there are symptoms of deficiency, much more than that amount is not likely to be useful.

In regard to all these matters, popular health literature has an important gadfly and informative role, but a very minor prescriptive one. By consulting such sources, a reader can keep abreast of the latest machinations of agribusiness, the drug firms, and the food industry. Readers can find guidance on the nutritional value of food groups and useful tidbits; an article may point out that pink grapefruit contains Vitamin A while white grapefruit does not, or that the nutritional value of brown and white eggs is the same. But when a nutritional cure is advocated for some condition, it is time to be wary.

If the vitamins and minerals to be added to the diet can be obtained through a reasonable choice of natural foods, there is little danger involved in following the suggestion. When this is not possible because of the huge amounts called for, the footnotes to the article must be consulted to locate the original research. Professional journals can be obtained or sent for through almost all state-university and public-library systems; and they are not as difficult to read as one might think. Often the recommendations will be found to be based on speculations arising from a small base of evidence. However, any treatment that appears promising can be brought to the attention of a physician. If such a research effort seems too much of a chore, then the original malady cannot be very serious and the risks of ingesting unusual quantities of vitamins and minerals are not justified. It must be remembered that the long-range effects of megadoses may be just as calamitous as those from medications. Only time will tell, and the era of massive vitamin intake is still in its infancy. Another consideration is to note that there are at least three distinct reasons for using any supplement: on a long- or short-term basis because for some odd reason the diet cannot provide it in adequate amounts; on a short-term basis as a medicine to treat a specific condition; and on a regular basis because of demonstrated need related to biochemical individuality.

Some health seekers, disgusted by supplements, medications, and technological gimmickry, turn to folk remedies as being somehow legitimized by virtue of their historical survival. Certainly much work remains to be done in systematizing knowledge developed in various folk traditions. Chemical analysis of plants used by folk healers has shown that some of them have genuine curative properties. In China, techniques like acupuncture are being evaluated for possible integration into a single body of medicine. But these are matters for highly trained professionals. By and large, sentiment aside, folk medicine has always been a trial-and-error procedure dependent on specific psychological, social, geographical, and dietary frameworks that cannot be easily replicated. It would be reckless to suppose that any single treatment come upon haphazardly and out of its original context is likely to effect a cure, particularly of a serious disease, that has eluded modern scientists. Throughout the world, the longest-living populations are precisely those which enjoy the most modern health services and the most advanced theoretical sciences. To believe otherwise is to cling to the mirage of a pristine health wisdom that never was.

The polar opposite of putting additional vitamins, minerals, and foods into the body is fasting—the temporary suspension of all fuel intake. Its advocates believe that fasting is ideal for periodically detoxifying the body. They argue that just as an animal that has been wounded will refrain from eating in order to allow the body to marshal all its reserves for healing, so cessation of eating will allow the body to concentrate on elimination of unwanted materials in the cells and arterial passages. Fasting is differentiated from starving in that starving connotes a breakdown in healthy tissues and vital organs, while fasting means that only fat reserves and nonessential tissue are affected.

A strong argument against fasting is that the longevity agenda will accomplish the same housecleaning benefits without fasting's several disadvantages. The foremost of these is that a few days of fasting will produce reactions of weakness, headache, and nausea. Even the ability to read comfortably is usually affected. There are serious dangers to maintaining the proper glucose level and threatened impairment of functions requiring water-soluble vitamins, minerals, and proteins not stored in the body. Consequently, most long fasts are conducted under supervision in hospital-like conditions marked by considerable periods of inactivity. Most religiously motivated fasts are candidly antihealth in that one of the objectives is the penitential mortification of the flesh.

Accepting the logic of the fasting advocates for a moment, there are a number of experiments which indicate that a semifast of about 500 calories a day is preferable to a total fast, in that the breakdown of unwanted bodily deposits proceeds at once without the accompanying trauma of closing down major systems.[7] A comparison can be made to steel mills, which are rarely shut down totally because of the enormous energy output needed to restart operations. On two major points there is no serious medical dispute: fasting is one of the most ineffective methods for long-term weight reduction, and prolonged fasts without proper supervision are dangerous.

Fasting appeals mainly to those who want a kind of quickie health fix that doesn't require surgery or medication. Denying the body its daily fuel also plays to the notion that instead of being the normal condition of the body, health is attainable only through discomfort and deprivation. Accounts of fasting for more than a day or so at a time (usually for religious reasons) are rarely encountered in biographies of the longevous or massive studies of those over 90.

People seeking to improve their health often resemble scorpions consuming their own tails. Beguiled by feats of modern medicine, too many overdiagnose and overmedicate their most trivial ailments. Others, aware of their poor diets, get lured into a complex balancing act of vitamin and mineral supplements. Still others seek out exotic foods and treatments. But most such measures to improve health actually imperil it. Taking into account the qualifications outlined earlier, a predominantly vegetarian diet with a high concentration of raw foods remains the best all-around bet for getting the proper amount of essential nutrients. The front line of health maintenance is no father than the nearest greengrocer or farmers' market.

11

THE LONGEVOUS PERSONALITY

> In every consideration of the medical art, the nature of the body must be regarded as a whole.
>
> —*Hippocrates*

The subtle complex of mental attitudes, behavioral patterns, and moral values that form an individual personality makes up the third critical sector of the longevity profile. Shaping a personality that is prolongevous is and no doubt will remain more art than science, for although some traits are readily identifiable as positive, few can be objectively measured in the way a given dietary or exercise item can be measured by caloric count or heartbeat. It is also apparent that many different personality types can be longevous as long as they do not aggravate the unavoidable physical and psychological stress of daily life.

One silly notion the longevity aspirant can dispose of at once is that the longevous are kindly, serene souls just this side of sainthood. They happen to be as caustic, self-centered, and jealous of their prerogatives as any other age group. Their lives will show the same incidence of marital discord, shrewd financial manipulations, and questionable moral judgments as those of the friends they have survived. Instead of having turned their backs on the world, the longevous have succeeded in overcoming, through one means or another, its most lethal challenges. If only by virtue of having lived to see their way of life vindicated by advanced age, they are likely to be unusually opinionated and strong-willed.

Not surprisingly, a key element in the longevous personality is the attitude toward time. The longevous have a marked preference for jobs that accommodate orderly, regular, and somewhat rhythmic daily patterns, and they have a distaste for those which involve constant anxiety. The longevous like to break down their work into doable segments of relatively short duration, allowing for periodic plateaus of accomplishment as well as vantage points from which to judge overall progress. If that progress is unsatisfactory, the schedule is apt to be shifted to the pace of work rather than the work speeded up to fulfill the original plan. Guided by entrenched personal standards and focused on well-defined goals, the longevous generally place a premium on quality of performance over speed or appeals to passing fashion.

The orderly routines preferred by the longevous tend to minimize bodily wear and tear while holding down the time lost to confusion, false starts, and panic. Breaking the work into doable segments means that there will be monophasic behavior—one major project at any given time receiving full concentration—rather than polyphasic behavior—a number of projects constantly competing for attention and inevitably pushing the body toward exhaustion in a pattern in which more and more energy is needed to accomplish less and less. Similarly, those who work late into the night or on split shifts have been shown to be among the least productive workers in terms of total output. By far the best model is one that is tuned to the natural cycles of the day and year, the prime example being the daily and seasonal schedule followed by farmers. Such routines mesh with the subtle biological rhythms of various bodily systems, such as the rising and falling of internal temperature and the pace at which various hormones are released.

An immediate benefit of a regularized rhythmic life-style is that it should produce good sleep, a condition essential for the body to refresh itself and to make internal repairs and adjustments. Invariably, longevous people report lifelong patterns of regular and satisfying sleep. Because of the same biochemical individuality that affects individual nutritional needs, there is such a wide variation in sleeping needs that it is best to ask not how long one has slept but how well. Most humans will be rested by from six to eight hours of sleep a night, with a few doing well on as little as four hours and a few requiring up to nine. People who take siestas in the middle of the day usually need fewer total hours of sleep. Otherwise, there is no apparent difference between those who take all their sleep at one time and those who divide it. Except for individuals recovering from an illness, regularly sleeping beyond nine hours should be as much a concern as insomnia or waking with a tired feeling. All three conditions may be symptomatic of serious psychological or physical illness, but more commonly they are the result of inferior scheduling or unresolved polyphasic behavior. Reaching for sleeping pills or stimulants only puts off a genuine resolution of the difficulty.

The antithesis of the longevous personality is the one that Drs. M. Friedman and R. H. Rosenman have identified in their book *Type A Behavior and Your Heart*[1] as being highly prone to heart attack. The Type A personality is characterized by a chronic sense of time urgency brought on by factors like polyphasic activities, unrealistic schedules, and constant deadlines, often self-imposed. Daily living patterns have a jerky or irregular nature. As the day draws on, the Type A is prone to falling further and further behind schedule, calling for frantic bursts of energy or resignation to working overtime. On a broader time scale, there are work on weekends, working holidays, and guilt about time

taken for play. A corollary attitude involves general insen-
sitivity to aesthetic values and little appreciation for
certain things' just being in the world, like a redwood
forest with trees centuries old which ought never be owned
or lumbered by private parties.

Frequently the Type A is thought of as a doer or a mover,
the perfect competitive type suitable for the business world.
This confuses mere motion with accomplishment, the wheel
spinning in place with one that can propel a vehicle forward.
The irritability and impatience of the Type A usually alienate
fellow workers to such a degree that although a fit of bullying
or an impassioned outburst may get short-term action, in the
long run lack of cooperation, lack of interest, and even
hostility from others become increasingly damaging to projects undertaken. One consequence of not breaking up work
into doable segments is the creation of a perpetual do-or-die
crisis ambiance that may culminate in emotional disaster.
The clenched fist, banging on the table, and shouting are
signs of a sinking psychological ship. More often than not,
the Type A has made the additional error of equating
efficiency with speed and quantity.

Numerous attempts have been made to measure the
damage done to the body by psychological and physical
stress. The most systematic work has been done by Hans
Selye, who has investigated the local and general adaptive
processes of the body. This has included examination of the
chemical alarm systems and responses in the central nervous
system and in glands such as the pituitary and adrenals.
Specific biological changes within the body are thought of as
barometers of how much the body is being stressed and how
successfully it is adapting.[2]

Selye believes physical stress is easier to cope with
because the cause is usually identifiable. The initial response
mechanism can be judged for effectiveness, and if it does not
work there is a renewed search for something that does. The
cause of psychological stress can be more elusive. Symptoms
like insomnia, stomach pains, or muscular tension are not

easily traceable to their psychological causes. While most people will understand that fighting rush-hour traffic in a car or being sandwiched in a crowded bus is likely to be stressful, fewer will appreciate that idleness can be just as dangerous. The body was made to work, and when it is idle, pent-up energy may cause a pervasive feeling of loginess. If this leads to more inactivity, the condition worsens. Finally, there are instances which are of a positive emotional nature but which require biological adaptation. Beginning a new school is one example. Momentary relief from stress of any kind can be obtained through various depressants, but in the long run they may only guarantee that when the stress reaches an intolerable level the residual damage will be far more severe than if the cause had been attended to sooner.

Strokes, ulcers, and migraines are only the visible tip of the stress iceberg. Selye believes that stress, influenced by dietary and exercise habits, is the leading cause of aging itself. The less change in the tissues and vital organs brought about by an adaptive response and the less stress to begin with, the slower the aging process. While not all stress can be avoided, and while there is a finite amount of adaptive capacity in the genetic bank, Selye is convinced that the average life-span could be increased tremendously if people lived in better harmony with natural laws. His suggestions for life extension mesh with the kind of moderation so often discerned in longevous profiles. For example, Selye writes that although the body must work vigorously in order to prosper, it is not constructed to take too much pressure on any one part, so that it makes prolongevous sense to diversify physical activity and to avoid pushing the organism to exhaustion. Muscular or mental activities that lead to definite solutions, such as those in monophasic behavior, prepare the body for sleep, while efforts that set up self-cycling tension or that lack a resolution promote stress.

Chronic stress can be caused by a major life pattern, such as the kind of exertion, eating, traveling, and sleeping dictated by one's occupation. Jobs that involve crowded facilities, sensory deprivation, constant crisis, or extreme isolation are not likely to be prolongevous. If eating is hurried, sleeping irregular, and travel a chore, there is need to question the basic life-style. The solution may be as drastic as changing jobs or living locations, or it may mean taking up formalized relaxation techniques such as deep breathing. In many instances, moderate adaptation responses such as walking an hour every evening will suffice. But failure to deal with stress or turning to drugs, alcohol, and tobacco for illusionary relief will cause rapid withdrawals on the genetic bank, culminating in premature aging.

The difference between what is stress and what is stimulation is often a matter of attitude. An illustration can be drawn from something as trivial as solving the Sunday crossword puzzle. Stress is set into motion if an individual imposes a time goal on the task and works at the solution as if it were a test of mental competence. Unable to find a Latin word that intersects with a Hindu god, a stress-prone person may get into a frenzy of dictionary research or call up the local librarian or friends for assistance. Physicians have observed that some persons become so emotionally distraught over crossword puzzles that their blood pressure rises to dangerous levels. As a result of these observations, many heart patients have been told to avoid activities of this kind. Yet gerontologists know that many longevous people regularly do crosswords and that the exercise helps keep their minds alert. The difference is that the longevous rarely impose a time limit on solving the puzzle and they get satisfaction from solving a quadrant of the puzzle or finding some difficult definition during any one sitting; they may take several days to complete the whole puzzle. If blanks occur where foreign words meet ancient deities, they are likely to see it as a failure of the puzzle maker as much as any lack of knowledge on their part. And if the puzzle doesn't appeal to them from the start, they can ignore it without feeling any threat to their self-esteem.

Related patterns can be found in attitudes toward play.

The longevous play in order to relax, while personality types most prone to stress damage turn play into tension. This is not to say that the longevous do not value skill building or that they avoid all competition. The Abkhasians love to race their horses and to play a form of polo. But they also enjoy breeding their horses, parading them, trading them, doing tricks with them, and just riding. The Type A personality identified by Friedman and Rosenman is likely to favor sports with one-to-one competition, to insist on the finest equipment available, and to seek out professional advice on honing their skills. Practice and playing of the sport become more items to stuff into the already crowded daily calendar. When drawn to jogging, the stress-prone types will be attracted by the marathon aspect, setting up complex training regimens in a new cycle of deadlines, tests, and anxiety. Getting up to marathon standards or winning at competition replaces recreation as the goal of the activity. Often the only emotional relief is that the sport is seen as part of a business or social commitment and thus is not wasted time and most certainly not idle play.

Individual response can determine whether or not a situation is stressful in many other ways. The predictability of the stress, the social context, and the amount of control involved affect the adaptive response. Most people who live near an elevated railway come not to "hear" or at least not to "mind" the rumble of the passing trains, even though some neighbors and almost all visitors may find them irritating. A child who needs to be disciplined may be extremely annoying to a father who insists on comparing his child with others who seem better-behaved, or the incident may be viewed as a creative part of parenting. A dripping faucet may ruin one woman's equilibrium if she is inept at home repairs, while another may take it in stride, using it as an opportunity to demonstrate mechanical skills not traditionally associated with her sex. Selling the family home may be heartbreaking to an elderly couple forced to the action by economic pressures or the sense that the structure is too large for them to keep up properly. The same situation may be viewed more positively by another couple who use the move as an opportunity to find housing that is less of a drain on resources, is closer to their children, or is better suited to their new pattern of social activities.

Many aspects of the prolongevous personality are thrown into high relief by the attitude toward retirement. In traditional agricultural societies like those of Soviet Georgia or in fishing towns like those on the Norfolk coast, it was the received knowledge of society that there would be no lessening of physical strength until sometime in the late 70s. From that point onward, the experience that had been gained by individuals was thought to qualify them as learned advisers to the family and community. In Sheringham this new counseling role was roughly equivalent to the former activist role, while in Georgia it had even higher prestige. For Georgian women, there was the added advantage of the erosion of restrictions based on sex. The assumption of long life in both societies put an age like 60 nearer to mid-life than to oncoming old age. In some parts of Abkhasia a ceremonial cane was awarded to individuals when they reached 90—not to aid them in walking, but to symbolize that they had finally become official elders.

Individuals in developed nations respond to entirely different expectations. The expectations of life are so constricted that retirement leaves one apparently at death's door. Usually the work ethic is so pervasive and family networks so frail that individuals, particularly males, feel that they *are* what they *do*. They come to feel that there is not much purpose to life if they cannot work. Thus, there is a high death rate in the years immediately following retirement. The psychological crisis is further intensified in societies that put a very high premium on youth, speed, and competition. Unlike the longevous Abkhasian, who embodies the highest virtues of the culture as taught by its opinion makers, the longevous American is likely to be a maverick, denying many of the values prized by contemporaries. In practical terms, longevous persons never truly retire. Either they have chosen jobs that do not require it, or they shift to new activities that are just as physically and intellectually demanding as their formal work had been.

The concept of retirement is based on economic, not biological, considerations. Since 1870, when the first national retirement program went into effect in Germany, the voluntary retirement age has drifted lower and lower, while the mandatory retirement age has been a matter of intense controversy. In some occupations, retirement is possible after a specific period of service, such as twenty or thirty years, so individuals entering the field at a young age may retire in their 40s or 50s.

The idea of insisting on mandatory retirement not linked to health or ability has been increasingly under fire in most nations. In the United States retired executives have been called upon by the government to act as advisers to novices trying to set up businesses with federal loans, and there has been pressure to allow those receiving Social Security to be able to work without losing any benefits—a practice followed in the Soviet Union, among other nations. The number of Americans who refuse conventional retirement continues to grow.

A change of interest can be more beneficial than rest. Three well-known contemporary Americans with widely different interests illustrate the new directions possible after age 70. Maggie Kuhn, at age 69, founded the Gray Panther organization to act as a political lobby for senior citizens. Her activities include regular appearances in the media and attendance at conferences in different parts of the nation. George B. Saunders, at age 68, founded a franchise system for fried chicken, using his private formula. It became one of the most successful fast-food outlet chains in the nation, and the distinctive white suit, goatee, and Southern charm of "Colonel" Saunders became familiar to millions of Americans. And I. F. Stone, a much-honored journalist, turned in his mid-70s to the translation of ancient Greek poetry.

Problems related to the age of retirement are usually discussed in the context of advanced technological societies, but an incident from recent Cuban history shows how the question is pertinent to any stage of economic development. In the first twenty years of the revolution that came to power in 1959, the emphasis had been on extending opportunities to youth and on getting all classes involved in reshaping and rebuilding the nation. About the only Cubans not asked to make sacrifices by donating labor to reconstruction were the old. It was a boast of revolutionaries that for the first time in Cuban history even a peasant could age without fear of economic hardship. Hence, the government was surprised to learn in 1976 of events in Baguano, a town of about five thousand inhabitants in what was formerly Oriente Province.[3]

During the previous year, a number of retired men in the town, mainly widowers who lived alone, felt isolated from the revolution and were displeased with the pace of change in their particular city. Although the mass media constantly reported what others were doing all over the island, the retirees were spending their days in idleness and didn't even have a decent place to meet for coffee and cards. Led by a man who was already caring for an infirm wife, they discussed the possibility of building a pavilion. At this time, the group involved 19 men, the youngest being 65, the eldest, 84. Most of the men had been sugar-mill workers and had never done construction work. After getting a halfhearted go-ahead from local officials, the retirees set about making plans and garnering materials. When they couldn't get certain pipes needed for the superstructure, they climbed over a wire fence and "liberated" a few samples from the local government warehouse. Finding the pipes suitable, they threatened to expose the manager of the warehouse, who had been hoarding materials for future projects, if he did not release what they needed. Through similar improvisations, they got other necessary materials. Just as the pavilion was nearing completion, the seating problem was solved when a lost truck carrying benches wandered into the town square. The driver, a stranger to the area, asked for directions to a building project. The retirees shepherded him to their cafeteria, where the benches were promptly unloaded and set in concrete.

Once the cafeteria was opened to the public, the central government moved to give the men official recognition. Following the rhetoric of the period, they were dubbed the Red Brigade of Pensioners. Growing in number to over 60 individuals, the group built a fish store, two parks, and some bus shelters. They then began to speak of rebuilding the town's burnt-out cinema. To do this they had to canvass the province for an architect to contribute a design and for experts to help them install a modern air-conditioning system. As the work on the theater got into high gear, a film team from Havana came to record the brigade's work and to document the new project. The images that make up this film illustrate the kind of changed attitudes one can find in retired people anywhere who find a new social role. Each man is seen working to ability, but it is real work, not make-believe work. One may be carrying but a single brick in each hand while another carries six. Another may roll building materials along the ground behind two others who are hauling similar materials in tandem. Most of the men say the brigade has been the most enjoyable work force they have ever been part of. One huge black man looks into the camera and says, "I really *love* this work." From being isolated individuals who were "tired of sleeping," the retirees have become a genuine community. They even play three-inning baseball games in their spare time.

The Cuban government doesn't quite know what to make of the initiative of the retirees. It does not want to appear to be putting pressure on other older people to do similar projects, yet it feels the experience should be shared. Local authorities have noted that the action of the retirees has galvanized their town, inspiring other social groups to similar community activities. At the pavilion, some of the original builders are now in charge of maintenance. Quite predictably, a physician assigned to monitor the men's health has found a marked improvement in their cardiorespiratory responses and a general improvement in their overall health.

If the longevous are atypical humans in their adamant refusal to retire from work even when they are financially able, they are prototypical in their living arrangements. The overwhelming majority have lived the greater part of their lives in a family unit, the percentage in the Soviet Union going over 98 percent. In the United States, at every age past 20, death rates are lower for those who are married than for those who are single, widowed, or divorced, the mortality for unmarried men living alone being the highest. Comparisons of Protestant and Roman Catholic clergy show that the Protestant clergy, who are allowed to marry, live longer.[4] The longevity factor, however, does not appear to be marriage itself so much as living in a situation that provides companionship and feelings of self-esteem, such as those described in the Cuban example. Returning to the Roman Catholic Church, students found better-than-average life-spans among 115,000 nuns who, although unmarried, lived in communal settings, had a high sense of social responsibility, and continued to work after age 65.[5] Cardinals of the Roman Catholic Church, like U.S. Supreme Court justices, have unusually long life-spans. Their zest for living is usually attributed to the power and honor associated with their high ecclesiastical office.

The companionship aspect of living arrangements is underscored by findings that feelings of loneliness often precede death and that long life among the old is usually associated with having at least one intimate friend of long standing. The loss of this friend often leads to the early death of the survivor. Retirement communities suffer from this phenomenon, as they are constantly recording deaths without having the full range of generations, which would include births, to redress the emotional balance. But such communities do have the advantage of keeping their inhabitants in touch with a wide social circle with many regularized community activities—quite a contrast to the nursing-home situation, where dependency and abandonment are the rule. The most prolongevous living arrangement, however, is a multigenerational household or community in which all adults have personal control over their private affairs.

The phenomenal marriage rate of the longevous sheds some light on their sexual practices—an area that has been little investigated, partly because of the modesty of older people in traditional societies and partly because even in modern nations, the subject has long been thought to be an improper one to bring up with women or the old. The puritan hangover about sex persisted in strength in the United States until the onset of the 1960s. Since then it has been easier to get data, but the materials remain sketchy. One study conducted by Duke University which covered over 200 men and women between the ages of 60 and 94 disclosed that 50 percent of them were enjoying sexual relations at the time of the interviews. Among octogenarians the rate was between 10 and 20 percent, with many stating that it was lack of suitable partners rather than lack of desire which prevented them from being sexually active. Other studies have indicated that the aged have far more liberal views on sexual matters than might be expected from stereotypes of the old or from the fact that anyone over 60 during the post–World War II period would have had his or her views shaped in a far less sexually permissive era. In general, frequency of sexual relations, while deminishing with age, was consistent with the strength of the sex drive throughout the particular individual's life; and couples usually did not totally cease having sexual relations until the health of one of them precluded it.[6] It was a common observation throughout the 1970s that the sexual activity and living arrangements found in retirement communities and at senior-citizen centers were not unlike those typical of other adults.

In the Soviet Union, the longevous describe their sexual lives as being regular, pleasant, but not excessive. Most accounts of the longevous which touch on sex report similar patterns; the males in particular state that regularity in sex is the key to maintaining potency until late in life. Despite claims of some men to sexual prowess after 90, and of some women to have given birth after 60, attempts to link old age and unusual fertility have been unsuccessful. Nonetheless, given the unusual physical and psychological vigor of those who become longevous and their marked penchant for marriage, it is logical to assume that their sexual activities are extended along with other vital interests. Longevous individuals frequently will credit successful marriages as the secret of their long life.

The self-esteem, flexibility, independence, and planning ability so marked in longevous persons are often tied to education. Statistics show that for white American males who were 22 years of age in 1900, a seven-year advantage in average life-span was enjoyed by those who graduated with honors from universities, and for most of the century, among white males, college graduates have usually outlived the eighth-grade dropouts by an average of five years.[7] The significance of the first finding is all the more dramatic as by age 22 the entire group of male babies born in 1878 yet still alive in 1900 had already survived the high mortality rates of infancy and childhood. This is slightly less important for the comparison between the college graduates and the eighth-grade dropouts. One factor at work, of course, is that the less well educated are likely to have more hazardous occupations, but the spread is too large and too pervasive to be accounted for solely on that basis. By and large, the professions all have longer average life-spans than other job categories. The major exceptions are farmers, who are long-living, and such professionals as journalists, air-traffic controllers, and accountants, whose work habits are either too stressful or too sedentary to promote long life. A survey of 6,000 males listed in the 1950–51 *Who's Who in America* found that they outlived other males handily.[8] Another study found that 1,000 corporate executives employed by the five hundred firms ranked by *Fortune* magazine as the most powerful in the United States were also long-living.[9] One of the positive correlations found in all these studies was that between the likelihood of long life and high measurable intelligence.

Findings of this sort do not indicate that only formal education will produce longevity or that self-esteem must be derived from prestigious occupations. If that were so, then women, generally excluded from higher education and the professions for so many centuries, would not be the larger longevity group. The prolongevous advantages of higher education and high social standing do indicate that long life is not linked to isolation from or rejection of conventional society.

The moderate spirit of the longevous so often commented upon tends to broaden rather than limit experience, for while many experiences are theoretically possible, not all are necessarily desirable. In the real world, in order to savor the nuances of any experience worth having, one has to make choices. Given two hours at a major museum, the prolongevous are going to choose a few galleries or a select list of items to concentrate on rather than trying to get a quick glance at everything, which, in effect, is to see nothing. Travel plans that promise seven countries in nine days are anathema. The prolongevous would not approve of youngsters who eat and watch television while studying, a polyphasic pattern in which the eating, viewing, and studying are all likely to be inferior. Nor are the prolongevous inclined to be the kind of social butterflies who make numerous phone calls and quickie visits and attend many obligatory social events to maintain a wide spectrum of acquaintances who will never develop into friends. In the end, by focusing on a limited number of experiences deemed highly desirable, the longevous succeed in doing, seeing, and feeling more than those who pride themselves on keeping all their options open. Those who refuse to make choices often end up like a pebble skimming off the surface of a pond; they are unable to make more than a fleeting impact anywhere, and everywhere they find only a mirror of the place they have just left.

In terms of geography, the most prolongevous locales are rural areas, with cooler climates having a slight advantage over warmer ones. The difference in average life-span between rural and urban areas in the United States is about five years. The investigation of 402 Americans over the age of 95 conducted by pollster George Gallup found that 74 percent of those participating had lived most of their lives on farms, in villages, or in small cities. Quite a few of the longevous lived within a few miles of their birthplace.[10] These findings are consistent with samplings taken in other nations.

Perhaps the least-understood aspect of the longevous personality, yet one of tremendous impact, is the expectation of health as the normal condition of life. While thinking won't make it so, it seems to help. Minimally, prolongevous convictions are needed to muster the determination to follow beneficial dietary, exercise, and living patterns. At age 75, it is imperative to consider the years that stretch to 100 as another quarter of life to be savored, not as the last sand in the time glass.

Just how powerful the benefits from a prolongevous mind-set may be is a matter of intense scientific scrutiny. The major focus has been on how mental attitudes affect the development of or recovery from specific diseases. An impetus to this line of investigation has been Hans Selye's work on stress which has already been referred to. It is speculated that if the physiological responses to stress are not resolved they may cause a disease, weaken the body's immunological system, or lessen the body's ability to fight a disease already contracted. Conversely, other physiological responses induced by positive psychological input might be able to increase the body's immunity to disease or aid it in resisting a disease already contracted. Setting up strict scientific measurements for this kind of research is extremely difficult, yet the field is promising, and the implications for longevity are tremendous.

The clearest examples of mind interacting with matter

are the kind of purely psychosomatic diseases that psychology has made us familiar with. A related phenomenon seen in all hospitals is that some patients on hearing they have a serious disease or must undergo painful treatments, seem to lose their will to live and fail to respond to treatment. The high mortality rates among people who have recently retired, who have just lost a spouse, and who live alone are in much the same category. Although the physical process by which emotions weaken the body is not precisely understood, there is little question that the interaction exists.

That the mind may be able to affect health positively is a more tenuous position, but there is some supportive evidence. Numerous studies have shown that death rates fall before major holidays. It appears that many who are extremely ill are somehow able to rally for one more major celebration or family reunion. Among individuals, it is common to find death some time after a birthday or important event rather than shortly before. In the area of "miracle" or "faith" cures, found in all major religions, investigators have discovered that after the ecstatic moment during which the first breakthrough to a cure takes place, a moment such as a lame person's suddenly walking, there will be a long period of recuperation in which recovery proceeds along predictable and gradual lines. A sore will not immediately disappear but will heal over a span of weeks or months. It is significant to note that among such cures there is no recorded incident of regeneration of limbs or correction of a genetically caused disease or condition. Even more interesting than religious cures (which are not easily verifiable) are controlled tests in various medical facilities which show that in some situations placebo cures are only slightly less effective than the medicinal cures for which they are substituted. The conclusion that could be drawn from these and similar findings is that the mind may be able to influence the body's ability to self-heal, either by rallying the natural curative mechanism already identified or by tapping as yet undetermined resources. It's been suggested, for example, that the endorphins, the body's own pain relievers, are released in response to placebos.

A number of approaches that attempt to deal with the response of the entire person have been grouped under the category of holistic medicine. Among the most respected medical workers in that field is Dr. O. Carl Simonton, whose specialty is cancer, the most dreaded of all modern diseases. Simonton was intrigued by the spontaneous remissions found in some cancer patients and in "cures" that resulted from drugs known to be generally ineffective. He wondered if some psychological profile might not make people more prone to cancer in the way a Type A profile made people more prone to heart disease. A comprehensive summation of his views appeared in *Getting Well Again*,[11] a book coauthored by Stephanie Matthews-Simonton and James Creighton. The authors present an impressive summary of placebo cures effected by different institutions and outline a theoretical model of how stress might cause malignancies. Another long section is devoted to mental techniques that might be used to fight cancer or to relieve the kind of stress they believe can lead to it and other maladies. The authors see their psychological work as a supplement to rather than as a replacement for standard cancer treatments. Simonton is a radiation oncologist.

A better-known example of how psychological attitudes may effect the cure of a difficult illness is the experience of Norman Cousins, editor for many years of *The Saturday Review*. In 1964, Cousins was struck down and crippled by ankylosing spondylitis, a severe collagen disease thought to be irreversible and incurable. Working closely with his physician, Cousins cured his ailment with an incredible will to recover and 25-gram daily doses of ascorbic acid. Pursuing the hypothesis that positive emotions might help in the curative process, Cousins chose to concentrate on laughter. He began by screening the films of the Marx Brothers and episodes of *Candid Camera*. His physician found that after hours of viewing the films, there were measurable positive physical reactions in the body. In order to continue with the unorthodox laugh therapy, Cousins had to move from the hospital to a hotel room, where he found the atmosphere much more congenial. Later he was to learn of a British study which showed that the survival rate of heart patients being treated in an intensive-care unit was no higher than that of those being treated at home—possible confirmation that a crisis atmosphere can nullify the impact of sophisticated technological support systems.[12]

Cousins first wrote about his recovery in *The New England Journal of Medicine* (December 23, 1976). After reprints of the article and follow-up essays had appeared, he published a full account of his experience, its aftermath, and possible implications in *Anatomy of an Illness.*[13] The original article of 1976 produced over three thousand letters from doctors commenting on every aspect of his recovery. This outpouring of professional concern indicated the enormous interest in the kind of issues Cousins, like Simonton and the holistic school, had raised. One might argue that it was the Vitamin C which had brought about the cure. In this respect, it is important to note that doctors who have used C to treat cancer patients generally believe it to be most effective in combination with standard treatments and that its impact is enhanced by the patient's belief that it will help. Along the same lines, Cousins has remarked that Dr. Jerome D. Frank of the Johns Hopkins University School of Medicine often refers to a study of 176 cases of cancer that were remitted without surgery, X-rays, or chemotherapy. Cousins concluded, "One wonders whether a powerful factor in those remissions may not have been the deep belief by the patients that they were going to recover and their equally deep conviction that their doctors also believed they were going to recover."[14]

The extent to which the mind can mobilize the rest of the organism to fight disease will not be known for quite some time; and it will take even longer to determine, if ever, exactly how mental attitudes affect overall health maintenance. But it is clear that psychologically depressed people are not likely candidates for long life and that people who set low expectation levels are self-programming premature aging. The prospects for immediate as well as long-term health are greatly enhanced by an understanding that attention to life-style greatly alleviates the noxious effects of stress. Rather than being a series of sacrifices, prolongevous habits activate the most natural, creative, and pleasant responses of the organism. Thinking longevously will not guarantee automatic entry to the century club, but like good exercise and dietary habits, it is one of the irreplaceable prerequisites.

12

THE TOXIC SOCIETY

> Most scientists agree that the over-
> whelming majority of cancers are
> environmentally caused. As such
> they are largely preventable. But the
> failure by the public, industry, and
> government to recognize this fact
> and act on it is why we have a
> cancer epidemic today, and why
> that epidemic may become even
> worse in the years ahead.
>
> *—Robert H. Boyle for*
> *the Environmental Defense Fund*
> *in* Malignant Neglect

An acidic rain has begun to fall. The nitrogen and sulfur oxides released into the atmosphere by various petrochemical processes have made some snow, hail, sleet, and rain as acidic as vinegar. The industrial Midwest of the American heartland has spawned acidic rains in New England and northern Canada, while the great industrial basins of Germany and Britain have caused acidic rains in the forests of Norway and Sweden. The Athenian Acropolis, symbol of Europe's loftiest dreaming, is so badly corroded by air pollutants that the Greek government is considering encasing it in a massive glass dome. Yet domes would hardly be practical for the fifty thousand high-altitude lakes in the Adirondacks and Canada that have been so poisoned that some plant life and entire fish populations have been decimated or totally eliminated. Snakelike domes stretching hundreds of miles would be needed to shield the meandering streams of Norway and

Sweden that are now lethal to salmon. As yet, the menace to human life from acïdic rain remains minimal, but the phenomenon is a sinister foretaste of environmental dangers to health and life that are uncontrollable by national, class, or individual action.[1]

Like poor eating habits and lack of exercise, environmental poisons may take decades to work their havoc. None are more fearsome in this respect than carcinogens, whose destructive force may gestate silently for ten to forty years before imperiling the host. With new synthetic chemicals and new sources of radiation being manufactured pell-mell, the developed nations are engaging in ecological brinksmanship whose slightest miscalculations could bring on terracidal reactions. If these threats to health and life continue to rise or even remain at present levels, the best-laid longevity plans will be seriously compromised. Self-interest dictates that the would-be longevous support, if not lead, the various movements aimed at environmental detoxification. At the same time, there are preventive measures which can modify the immediate personal dangers considerably.

As recently as the 1860s, a nation like the United States could rightly boast of the quality of its environment. The industrialization which began in earnest shortly thereafter adversely changed the situation, but massive environmental deterioration did not commence until the introduction of petrochemicals in the 1930s and the dawn of the nuclear age in the 1940s. By the 1970s, the body of every American contained residues of some of the quarter-million industrial chemicals in use. Every one of the thousands of synthetic chemicals was a substance that could not be found in nature and whose interaction with life forms could be only a guesstimate.

The center of toxicity is the industrial workplace.[2] Irrefutable research has established the link between cancers and working with substances like vinyl chloride, asbestos, industrial dyes, chromates, nickel, uranium, and glass fibers.

More specifically, previously rare cancers can be tied to precise substances. Mesothelemia with asbestos, angiosarcoma of the liver with vinyl chloride and polyvinyl chloride, and oat-cell carcinoma with bis-chlormethyl ether are three examples. The linkage of black lung with coal mining and brown lung with textile weaving also is beyond scientific dispute. Where such clear and present dangers exist in the workplace, the would-be longevous have no option but to switch to other industries and to remove their residences from proximity to toxic workplaces. A drastic response of this kind is dictated by the pattern of attempts to bring industrial pollution under control, a history marked by the unwillingness of the companies to face up to the danger of the processes they have set in motion and by the slowness of government in establishing adequate safeguards for workers or the public.

The negative properties of the most dangerous substances usually were known decades before effective regulation. Vinyl chloride's link to cancer was first suspected in the late 1940s; the dangers of industrial dyes were known in the 1890s; and the various effects of asbestos, established conclusively at the turn of the century, were described by physicians in ancient Greece. In spite of this history, all three were used with abandon until well into the 1970s; and although the amount of exposure considered safe has been consistently lowered, corporate managers and their medical experts have stubbornly defended the adequacy of each new and lower safety threshold. In most instances, regulation would not have been imposed if unions representing the affected workers had not financed medical studies of their own and publicized the results in the mass media. Arguments over acceptable standards of exposure have dragged on for years while the substances continue to produce incalculable numbers of premature deaths, painful diseases, and sterility. The burden of proof has always been on the victims, and even when they have been proved to be aggrieved parties, the

responsible manufacturer has rarely made financial settlements—even though no payment can really compensate for
loss of life or catastrophic illness.

Given these realities, workers dealing with chemicals of
any kind stand in danger of developing cancer as one of their
"fringe benefits" of employment. To prevent this, they must
have their unions finance independent studies of every
substance to which they are exposed. When there is any
doubt about safety, the margin of error must be on the side of
prudence. If safety equipment and special procedures are
suggested by the manufacturer, they should be followed to
the letter. Legislation also must be developed to make
corporations liable for environmental damage and personal
injuries, even if the problem stems from honest miscalculations. If there is conscious deception regarding health hazards, criminal charges of the kind that would apply to any
premeditated poisoning should be imposed. A responsible
step in this area was taken in 1979 when the Nuclear
Regulatory Commission proposed to fine Consumers Power
Company of Jackson, Michigan, $450,000 because the utility
neglected for *eighteen months* to close the valve on a 4-inch
pipe leading into its reactor containment building.[3] No
radioactivity escaped, but if there had been an accident of the
type that occurred at Three Mile Island the results would
have been catastrophic. The proposed fine was the largest in
the NRC's history and served as a warning of the public's
growing intolerance of negligent safety procedures in industry. Only such stringent measures can make compliance with
environmental regulations cost-effective for affluent pollu-
ters, and absolutely imperative for managers, researchers, and
other responsible individuals. When the acidic rains become
lethal to human life, it will be too late to ask which firms or
individuals were responsible.

Industrial planners habitually save money for their firms
by using the environment as a garbage dump. They release
dangerous by-products into waterways, push them out of
smokestacks into the air, and allow them to seep into the

soil. The eventual victims of this pollution may be hundreds or thousands of miles downriver or downwind, making it difficult to pin the pollution tail on the responsible donkey. The public needs to understand that cancer results when there are continuous insults to the body by noxious chemicals. Even minute quantities may cause the disease, but the risks definitely increase with the amount and time of exposure. Thus it does not seem purely coincidental that wherever there is a concentration of petrochemical industries there is a cancer hot spot. The most prominent example is the infamous cancer alley of New Jersey which runs along the industrial complex bordering the New Jersey Turnpike. In addition to the phenomenal cancer rates found in some factories located in that corridor, communities on Staten Island and in Brooklyn, separated from the source of contamination by miles of water, also are affected because of the prevailing westerly winds.

Risks from the air, however, are most serious in metropolises where industrial wastes are trapped by skyscrapers and where automobile exhausts add to the toxic overload. Although the petrochemical smog of Los Angeles is prototypical of this category, numerous cities have similar problems. One defensive measure has been to have health bureaus alert the public when the air quality is inferior. If such an alarm is given, no would-be longevous person and certainly no one with a chronic heart or respiratory disease should be out of doors more than absolutely necessary. At such times strenuous work or exercise does not demonstrate hardiness so much as foolhardiness. The best course is to gain the protection of air conditioning, which filters out many pollutants. Should one's city of residence have many days with unsatisfactory air quality, relocation must be considered. Air is not a luxury like a banana cream pie; it contains the oxygen that is vital if cells are to maintain the organism for the one hundred plus years of life for which it is intended.

Sinister as the air-pollution problem is, most cities have experienced considerable improvement in their air quality throughout the 1970s. In contrast, there has been only the genesis of an effective reaction to a far more potent atmospheric danger: exposure to tobacco smoke. Although the smoker is the primary victim, any small room with even one person smoking in it will have a higher level of carbon monoxide, carcinogens, and toxins than the entrance to most factories. The dangers to longevity are acute. According to a follow-up report of the Surgeon General released in 1979, a two-pack-a-day habit will reduce the smoker's lifetime by from eight to nine years and will increase the overall death risk at every age by about 70 percent. A survey issued later in the same year by the State Mutual Assurance Company of America independently confirmed the government's conclusion. Based on 100,000 policyholders, the insurance report found that at every age after 20, smokers had at least double the mortality rate of nonsmokers and that for certain diseases such as lung cancer the risk was as much as 15 times as great. The average life-span of the policyholders who smoked was from seven to eight years less than for nonsmokers. The company backed its findings by offering lower premiums to nonsmokers. These reports of the Surgeon General and State Mutual were in line with worldwide health research on smoking that had been ongoing for at least twenty years; the first scientific paper linking tobacco and cancer dates to British studies done in 1761.

One effect of smoking not widely appreciated is its devastating synergistic effect in combination with toxins. An asbestos worker has 16 times as great a probability of developing cancer as the average American, but if the asbestos worker also smokes, the probability leaps to 60. Analysis of death rates among urban dwellers indicates that those who do not smoke do not have a significantly higher incidence of various respiratory diseases than those who live in rural areas, but urban dwellers who do smoke do. One explanation for this is the synergistic interaction of air pollutants and tobacco smoke. This interpretation is supported by findings that the most polluted cities do not have the highest rates of lung cancer and that there is not much difference between lifelong residents of cities and recent arrivals. Furthermore, there is considerable difference between males and females and between manual workers and professionals. In each case the group with the greater percentage of smokers has a far greater incidence of respiratory disease.

During the 1970s lung cancer was the leader in cancer deaths for men and third for women. Given that 85 percent of lung cancer is linked to smokers and a good portion of the remainder to identifiable workplace risk, it can be seen that a disease which killed approximately 100,000 persons annually was being caused primarily by tobacco smoke, with air pollution mainly a synergistic factor. The urgency of these data was underscored when the Surgeon General announced that, owing to the continued increase in smoking among women, it was projected that by 1983 lung cancer would be the major cancer among females as well as males.

Other negative aspects of smoking can be seen in the American Cancer Society studies which show that if one smokes only a pack of cigarettes a day, in addition to the chance that lung cancer will increase by 684 percent, the chance for cancer of the mouth increased 890 percent, for cancer of the larynx 709 percent, for cancer of the esophagus 317 percent, for cancer of the bladder 100 percent, and for cancer of the pancreas 169 percent. The use of filter tips and low-tar cigarettes reduced the odds, but such gains were lost if the number of cigarettes smoked increased because of the illusion of safety. Pipe smokers and cigar smokers also ran lower risks, but compared with nonsmokers the chances for cancer of the lung were 120 percent higher, for cancer of the mouth 150 percent, and for cancer of the larynx 200 percent. For cancer of the bladder, the risk was 100 percent greater for pipe smokers and 400 percent greater for cigar smokers.[4]

At least eight carcinogens have been found in tobacco smoke, and there is a positive correlation between higher doses and higher probability of disease. The Surgeon General's reports further indicate that coronary disease is even more likely than lung cancer and that there is a much higher risk of lung disorders such as emphysema. The one bright note is that the body is capable of overcoming some of the damage. If even a heavy smoker of two packs a day quits, in the course of fifteen years the average life expectancy and the chance of developing degenerative diseases gradually move to those of nonsmokers.

In spite of this overwhelming evidence, the United States, like other nations, has refused to treat tobacco as it would treat a dangerous microbe which murdered more than a million people every decade. Tobacco firms are allowed to propagandize their wares in mass media, and the government continues to subsidize many marginal growers who might otherwise be forced into bankruptcy. Regulation of smoking in public places is vigorously opposed by a combination of economic interests and addicts who believe smoking is something of an inalienable right even though it endangers the health of others. It is hard to remember, at times, that smokers are not only a minority of the adult population, but a declining minority.

Some smokers are comforted by the idea that breathing city air is equivalent to smoking. This error is based on misinterpretation of studies such as the one which found that a person standing in Manhattan's Herald Square for twenty-four hours would be exposed to the same amount of pollutants as found in two packs of cigarettes. One must realize not only that no one would stand in Herald Square for twenty-four hours, but that the intersection is far from typical: it is the crossroads of three major traffic arteries (34th Street, Broadway, and the Avenue of the Americas), there are many tall structures (including the Empire State Building) in the vicinity, and it is affected by the adjacent garment district and department stores, which have an unusually high concentration of idling truck traffic. Even so, the pollutants in this atypical area would be randomly distributed throughout the air, while those in a cigarette are highly concentrated, being heaviest exactly in that portion which enters the mouth. The dangers for a Herald Square pedestrian are potential; the ones for a smoker, actual. Moreover, when breathed through the nose, the natural filtering system of the body, some pollutants will be kept from entering the lungs. In contrast, tobacco smoke is deliberately inhaled directly into the lungs. Because of this, exhaled smoke, which has left many of its poisons inside the smoker's body, is less dangerous than undiluted smoke from a burning cigarette. Smokers still enamored of the Herald Square study also must face the fact that whatever dangers do exist in such locations are geometrically higher for them because of the synergistic syndrome and because of accelerating risks that result from an increased total intake of carcinogens.

By now it should go without saying that no one remotely interested in longevity will smoke, and that he or she will be as vigorous as possible in not allowing smoking in his or her presence. Without relinquishing concern for general air quality, the would-be longevous must put a priority on eliminating the number one cause of the number one cancer, a cause that is far easier to control than the atmosphere of a major city or of an industrial complex. In *Preventing Cancer*, Dr. Elizabeth Whelan has put it succinctly:

> Ironically, many people who are worried about the adverse effects of air pollution overlook the most obvious form that we come in contact with: one cigarette smoker, in a matter of minutes, can fill a closed room with higher concentrations of the carcinogen benzo (a) pyrene than are found in the most polluted city air in the world. If you are worried about the effects of air pollution on your lungs, your best bet would be to ban smoking in offices and public places.[5]

Dr. Whelan also offers an interesting analysis of the growth of cancer in the United States during the twentieth century. She calculates that when respiratory cancers, which were extremely rare in 1900, are eliminated from the statistics, the overall cancer rate for men has declined and the rate for women is nearly stable. Whelan then points out that breast and colonic cancers are highly influenced by the fat-heavy American diet. Though we may not necessarily accept her contention that it is fat consumption per se and not toxic substances accompanying fatty foods which are the nexus of the problem, her reasoning leads to the conclusion that the major contributing causes to the top three cancer killers for women (breast cancer, colonic cancers, and lung cancer) and the two top cancer killers for men (lung cancer and colonic cancers) are tobacco smoking and fat-laden diets. This analysis offers substantial support for two pillars of the longevity agenda: no smoking and a low-fat diet.[6]

When lung cancer is included in cancer statistics, the rise in the rate of cancer from 1968 through 1978 is 2.5 percent or 12 percent, depending on the method of calculation. The first figure would indicate only the mildest increase, especially in light of declining deaths due to cardiovascular diseases, but the second could signal the onset of an epidemic. The larger figure of 12 percent is a recording of the actual cancer deaths in the total population. The 2.5-percent increase is derived by "adjusting" of the increases for age, a practice established by the American Cancer Society and then picked up by the National Center for Health Statistics (Department of Health, Education and Welfare). This "adjustment" is based on the assumption that cancer is associated with biological aging. If this were true, older people would "naturally" have more cancers. It would then follow that since the percentage of the American population which is older is growing, it would be necessary to adjust statistics in order for different time periods to be compared without the influence of the changed age structures.

But the assumption that cancer is due to the aging process is dubious. In societies where there are no high cancer rates, the increase with age is not significant. Intercultural studies show that sites for cancers shift with migration, so that Japanese in Japan have one set of cancers and Japanese-Americans have another without age's being a factor. Sexual differences show the same pattern. Women in cultures with high breast-cancer rates have one incidence curve and women in societies without high breast cancer have quite another.[7] Studies of isolated groups with high cancer rates usually report a specific type or types of cancer associated with a specific cause—a pattern of the kind found in workplace cancers and one not influenced by age. Even within the United States, cancer rates fall off after the 80th year, when biological defenses presumably would be increasingly weaker.

A far more credible explanation for cancer in older populations living in toxic societies is that they have simply lived long enough to survive the ten-to-forty-year latency period between cancer insult and malignancy. This certainly seems to be true for lung cancer, where an increase or decrease in smoking in any identifiable segment of the population is followed in ten to twenty years by a corresponding increase or decrease in the disease. On balance, the practice of adjusting cancer rates for age appears to be little more than a statistical sleight of hand which makes some cancers disappear from the charts and transmutes probable environmental cancers into unlikely genetic ones. This appears to be yet another instance in which medicrats have come to the assistance of industry through statistics and projections that minimize the effects of pollution and work to assuage public concern.[8]

Other cancer statistical trends augur poorly for the future. One is that cancer has become the number two killer among children between the ages of 5 and 14 and that excepting influenza deaths between the ages of 1 and 4, cancer is the number one killer disease for males and females from birth to age 25.[9] Among those from 25 to 44, cancer is the leading cause of death for females and the third leading killer of males, trailing accidents and heart diseases. This pattern does not suggest the profile of a disease of old age.

Statistics also show that since the 1950s the more than century-long rise in the average life-span has all but stagnated. In spite of numerous medical advances since that time, the pluses and minuses of living in advanced technological societies have begun to cancel out one another. No one has yet dared to argue that environmental pollution should be added to the credit side of the longevity ledger. The prognosis for the rest of the century is further clouded by the fact that prior to the 1940s the petrochemical industry was still in its infancy and suffering through the stagnation of the Great Depression. Toxic exposure for the general public remained limited. Assuming the usual latency periods, the mortality impact of the petrochemical boom after 1950 may not become pronounced until the 1980s and '90s when the first humans with lifelong exposures to high dosages of synthetic chemicals and background radiation come into their middle years.

Public awareness of environmental health hazards is not novel. Some of the most popular nineteenth-century authors made reference to the fact that hatters were subject to brain damage because of the mercury used to tan furs (Lewis Carroll) and that chimney sweeps were prone to respiratory diseases (Charles Dickens). A host of writers addressed the maladies found among miners. What is unusual in the twentieth century is that distinctions between workplace risk and general risk are being obliterated. The high rate of cancer among naval-yard employees working with asbestos takes on new urgency when do-it-yourselfers trying to improve their living spaces find themselves confronted with asbestos insulation or when parents disturbed by alarming cancer rates in grade-school children find them linked to asbestos materials used in school construction. Millions more are shocked to discover that many hand-held hair dryers are lined with thin asbestos shields which can easily flake into the stream of hot air being blown around their faces or that some brands of electric toasters have asbestos liners in proximity to the bread being prepared for breakfast. Automobile mechanics can only wonder if the asbestos used in brake linings isn't as dangerous to them as to the original production workers who assembled them at the cost of extremely high rates of lung disease.

Asbestos is not an isolated example. Other household manifestations of workplace toxins would include the petrochemical insect-killing strips which work by poisoning the atmosphere, glass-fiber draperies which may release splinters into the air, and miracle cleaners, paint strippers, and glues which do their work through chemical reactions that may injure the body. Considerable controversy also surrounds the use of various plastics to wrap and store food because of the possibility that petrochemicals may leach into the food. It has been found, for example, that lemon and tea will interact with a polystyrene cup in a manner that dissolves the container and releases carcinogenic material into the tea.[10] Keeping abreast of these hundreds of disputes is a hopeless task for any individual. Reliance on as many natural materials as possible for household wares and furnishings is an excellent defensive measure, but ultimately the only long-term solution is regulating petrochemicals at the point of production.

Among the longer-range hazards to health that begin in the workplace and spread to the home are fluorocarbons. The problem with these compounds is that they deplete the protective ozone layer in the earth's atmosphere. By the end of the century, if use continues at the present level, the ozone layer will be lessened by 15 percent, greatly increasing the incidence of human skin cancer and setting the stage for unpredictable climatic changes. In the United States, until an aroused environmental movement forced a partial ban, fluorocarbons were found in most aerosol spray cans used in the home. Fluorocarbons are still used as refrigerants throughout industry. Worldwide, they are found in numerous household and industrial products.

A dangerous escalation of environmental dangers is occurring with the introduction of nuclear power as a major energy source. Three hazards are involved: the possibility of explosions, the probability of accidents, and the certainty of radioactive waste. These perils stem from the phenomenon that any exposure to radiation is harmful to the human body. As Nobel Laureate George Wald has said, "Every dose is an overdose . . . A little radiation does a little harm, a lot does more harm."[11] Natural sources of radiation are not exceptions to this rule. Navajo Indians working as uranium miners suffer epidemic-level cancer rates, and Yemenis who live near radioactive thorium sands have 25-percent higher rates of mental retardation than their neighbors. On the military front, major nuclear powers, such as the United States and the Soviet Union, are so aware of the dangers of atmospheric poisoning that they have voluntarily limited themselves to underground testing of their nuclear weapons and have tried to make this a universal practice. Most of the developing atomic powers have not yet seen fit to follow their lead, and every time such a nation makes an atmospheric test, radioactive clouds float around the world with no one able to predict upon which unlucky nation the radioactive fallout will descend.

Nuclear proponents are correct in stating that the possibility of an explosion at an energy plant is remote; but the possibility is not zero, and the destruction would be far greater than that seen at Hiroshima or Nagasaki. Accidents are of an entirely different probability order. Human error, equipment malfunctioning, aging facilities, and natural disasters such as earthquakes make every nuclear plant an accident waiting to happen. The Three Mile Island crisis of 1979 was only the most serious of numerous power-plant accidents; its distinction was to demonstrate with awesome drama the Faustian risk in putting nuclear time bombs in even moderately populated areas. Radioactive steam had to be released repeatedly as problem after problem plagued attempts to cool off the reactor, and once the meltdown threat had been averted, there remained enormous decontamination and waste problems.

Because low-level radiation does not kill instantly in the

manner of a bullet through the heart, the Three Mile Island utility could boast that not one person had been killed by the accident. But it will take decades to determine the validity of that assertion. In Utah and other areas where there had been atmospheric atomic testing the doubling and tripling of cancer rates did not become evident for twenty years, and the actual impact can never be determined. To prove that any particular cancer or birth defect is linked to a particular exposure is extremely difficult. Attorneys in liability cases must argue statistical probabilities. Numerous distortions result when people have moved out of an exposed area while others are moving in, making an accounting of exposure levels nearly impossible. These problems are compounded by the reluctance of those responsible for the contamination to determine the effects of their acts or even to be candid about the amount of exposure created. If guiltless, they have gained little at great expense; if guilty, they have opened themselves to litigation. In this respect the government has a worse record than private concerns, having suppressed warnings of its specialists and having deliberately lied to the public about the dangers involved in nuclear testing. The most callous act was the dispatch of Army units into radioactive zones in the 1950s in a bravura effort to demonstrate safety. Cancer rates among the exposed men have been far above the statistical norms, yet the afflicted soldiers have found it impossible to obtain government compensation. The same situation is likely to hold true for the eventual victims of the Three Mile Island incident and other accidents.

Thornier dilemmas revolve around the problem of nuclear waste. Until a method is found to deradiate wastes, the radioactive life-span of wastes is measurable in tens of thousands of years. At present, the most common method of control is to encase the material in lead containers and bury them in tunnels or caves. Such procedures place enormous faith in the longevity of the shielding and in the ability to safely move the wastes to dump sites. This is no one-time problem. The more nuclear plants there are, the faster the waste materials will accumulate. Assuming that there will be a continued use of radioactive substances for medical purposes and for military defense, disposal is an endless problem.

Without becoming hysterical over the safety issue, the would-be longevous will not want to live within a hundred miles of any nuclear plant or storage area, and most certainly not downwind or downriver from either. They also will be concerned about the routes and methods used to transport radioactive waste to the storage areas. As with other nuclear problems, the involved utilities are not to be counted on for candor or restraint. Until stopped by local political pressure, utilities were moving atomic wastes through the residential streets of New York City, the most densely populated area of the United States. The would-be longevous can do without exposure to risk of this sort or any of the other risks involved with nuclear power. The advantages nuclear power has over fossil fuels are chimerical, being at best the difference between environmental slavery and environmental serfdom. The national treasure and scientific expertise would be better directed toward developing technologies based on nonpolluting solar, wind, and tidal power, with nuclear input held to a minimum if utilized at all. Such a course would begin to make the world of technology compatible with the world of biology and begin the eradication of cancer and other diseases of industrial development.

The hazards of radiation to longevity are not limited to a few nuclear plants any more than petrochemical contamination is limited to the workplace. Without fanfare, common household items have become sources of radiation. One of these items is the microwave oven, which sits in the heart of the kitchen and may emit radiation if defective. Smoke-detector alarms that feature ionized particles are so perilous that the installation instructions warn that when the detector is dismantled it should not be discarded in a regular garbage dump—a warning most likely to be long forgotten by a second or third occupant of the premises. Even more common than microwave ovens and smoke detectors with ionized particles are devices with radium dials and paints that glow in the dark. The amount of radiation exposure involved from these household items is small, but as with additives in foods, a growing number of small exposures may add up to a major risk.

Despite assurances from manufacturers, the safety thresholds for X-rays, background radiation, and ultraviolet radiation of the type found in sunlamps are very much in doubt. The accepted annual X-ray exposure level during the 1970s was fixed at 5 rems per year, but at decade's end a special committee of the National Academy of Sciences suggested that the level should be lowered to .5 rems, the amount of exposure in a single chest X-ray. Even this vast difference pales when one realizes that the Soviet standard for microwave exposure is 10 microwatts per square centimeter while the U.S. standard is a full thousand times as great, or 10,000 microwatts per square centimeter. Such questions about safety are far from academic, affecting as they do the life of every citizen. Adding to the risk with radioactive household appliances defies common sense.

Government control over sources of radiation remains a matter of great anxiety. Four stories that surfaced late in 1979 illustrate the laxity and outright deception that have been typical for decades. In Denver, workers at the Robinson Brick & Tile Company were stunned to learn that the factory where some had been working for years had been built on a former (1914–17) dump site of the National Radium Institute.[13] In the Southeast, some one hundred thousand dwellings were found to have been built with concrete blocks made from radioactive slag sold to construction companies by the Tennessee Valley Authority.[13] In Los Angeles, Atomics International admitted that in 1959 it had released radioactive gases over the San Fernando Valley after a serious accident at an experimental nuclear plant.[14] And in Washington, D.C., a report suppressed for twenty-six years finally revealed that 4,200 sheep that had died in Utah in 1953, after exposure to a 24-kiloton blast, had been severely radiated.

Their thyroid glands showed a concentration of radioactivity that surpassed the maximum permissible concentrations for humans by from 200 to 1,000 times.[15] These four incidents had numerous counterparts throughout the nation. To them could be added the disputes over the widespread use of radioisotopes and CAT scanners (computerized axial tomography) as diagnostic tools in medicine. People concerned about exposure levels pointed out that medical history is replete with high mortality rates among researchers, doctors, nurses, and patients due to ignorance of or overly optimistic estimates of permissible exposure levels.

This combination of pure bungling, deliberate cover-up, and scientific arrogance about carcinogens and toxins has created a society in which the most intimate items must be viewed skeptically. Skin irritations frequently are the consequence of the chemicals used in cosmetics, synthetic fabrics, and toiletry items. Cosmetics that are applied in the vicinity of the eye, nose, and mouth should be chosen with extreme care; and it is an excellent practice to forgo colored or printed facial or toilet tissues for undyed white. The most dangerous product line so far identified in this category is hair dyes. Almost all permanent hair dyes and most tints, rinses, and semipermanent dyes contain carcinogens. Unless the consumer is certain this is not the case, such products should be avoided, as the carcinogens can be absorbed into the body through hair follicles. Henna, a plant product whose highlighting and tinting effects last several weeks, can serve as a noncarcinogenic substitute.

A toxin that works much faster and is even deadlier than radiation and the carcinogens in dyes is dioxin, a substance used in herbicides and defoliants. This poison first came to public attention at the time of the war in Vietnam. From 1962 to 1971, 10.6 million gallons of Agent Orange, a defoliant containing dioxin, were sprayed over the Vietnamese jungles in an effort to deprive guerrilla forces of cover. Over 1,000 Americans took part in the spraying and 6,000 more were exposed to it. The number of Vietnamese exposed is undetermined, but probably considerably higher. The difficulty with dioxin is that in addition to defoliating trees and killing pests, it has severe adverse effects on the human body, causing cancers, miscarriages, and birth defects. How long it is retained in the soil in a dangerous state is not known.

American servicemen who were exposed to dioxin have experienced extremely high rates of cancer, including rare brain tumors, high mortality rates, and high percentages of birth defects among their children. Officials in Vietnam report similar findings. The U.S. military has refused to admit any connection with its use of dioxin and has shied away from moral culpability in what amounts to chemical warfare. In an effort to determine responsibility, some veterans have litigated in the American courts. Five manufacturers of the defoliant have replied with legal briefs in which they accuse the government of acting negligently and recklessly. They state that the government failed to notify soldiers of the hazards of dioxin, failed to instruct them in proper handling methods, and failed to provide medical assistance when needed.

The controversy over the use of dioxin in Vietnam is just one example of human exposure to the substance. Silvex, a spray containing dioxin, has been used extensively in reforestation projects in Oregon, where dioxin has subsequently been linked to miscarriages and other health problems. Power companies throughout the nation have used dioxin to keep down unwanted vegetation around their utility poles. They and the manufacturers insist that when used with the recommended safeguards, dioxin is useful and safe.

Individuals living in areas exposed to dioxin sprays have become increasingly skeptical of corporate and governmental statements that their health is being adequately protected. They might be even more uneasy if they knew about the toxic aftermath of a chemical explosion which released dioxin and other chemicals into the environment of Seveso,

Italy, in 1976. The danger was so great that the most
contaminated zone had to be evacuated. Women in the first
three months of pregnancy are prohibited from living in
another, less-contaminated zone, and children under 12 are
barred during daytime hours. All animals in the district have
been slaughtered, some 600 children have developed skin
diseases, and there has been an increase in birth defects.
Committees investigating the explosion uncovered a familiar
pattern: Hoffman–La Roche, the company involved, had
attempted, at the beginning, to minimize the dangers, and the
local health officials had not been prompt in seeking outside
assistance. Eventually, Hoffman–La Roche paid $23 million
in damages to individuals and companies and another $54
million to various branches of the Italian government for
emergency and cleanup operations.

Still another toxic source is the water faucet. One of the
great leaps forward in life extension during the nineteenth
century was purification of drinking-water supplies, but
yesteryear's source of infectious diseases may be today's
source of environmental ones. Auto plants in Michigan
annually dump nearly fifty thousand pounds of phosphorus
into the Detroit River, and steel mills in Ohio pollute the
Cuyahoga with 137.5 tons of solids and 182,200 pounds of
sulfur, chlorine, phenol, cyanide, ammonia, magnesium,
iron, and oil. This sort of dumping is found in every
American waterway. Consequently, it is not surprising that a
study of eighty-eight counties in Ohio showed that death
from cancers of the digestive tract were much higher in areas
served by surface water than in those using wells. In New
Orleans, where the Mississippi flows toward the Gulf of
Mexico carrying the agricultural and industrial toxins of
more than a dozen states, cancers of the kidney, bladder, and
urinary tract are abnormally high. From the Hudson to the
Columbia the story is the same: the mighty rivers of America
have become so severely polluted that the purification systems of many cities are no longer adequate to deal with the
problem. From 1940 to 1960, there were 228 outbreaks of

poisoning due to the water supply; but as in most pollution problems, the cause-and-effect relationship between contaminant and diseases was impossible to document with precision because of time lapses, population shifts, and multiple causes of degenerative diseases.

Residents of small towns and country dwellers are not necessarily free of water-pollution woes. The most modest factory can affect an underground water table from which wells draw. Any strange odor or foaming in a stream or rivulet warrants immediate investigation. Assistance is available from the Environmental Protection Agency and local public-health officers. Should the water prove to be less than satisfactory, using bottled water provided by a responsible concern takes care of the major dangers. Filtration devices for water taps also can be considered, but a good consumer's guide should be used, as many of the items for sale are useless or dangerous.[16]

Water contamination is often due to poorly supervised or illegal chemical dump sites where toxins leach into the soil. Of equal concern at such sites is the dangerous mixture of wastes. If the storage drums should break or rust through, the resulting chemical interactions can produce fires, explosions, and release of lethal gases. Additional public risk results when haulers paid to transport wastes to legal dumps decide to pocket the fees and dump the load into a vacant city lot or secluded country area. What the driver considers a minor infraction of the law is much closer to a capital crime; but until the punishments involved bring home the gravity of the offense, illegal dumping and slipshod supervision of dumps will persist. Just like nuclear power plants, dump sites are environmental time bombs.

The Environmental Protection Agency has estimated that a general cleanup of dump sites would cost over $50 billion—still another example of how petrochemical thrift is a farce, the cost simply being shifted from the private to the public sector. The consequences of not taking action are visible in the disaster that occurred in the Love Canal area near Niagara Falls, New York. Here, thousands of people had to be permanently resettled and nearly eight hundred homes had to be purchased by the state when the immediate threat to life and health from a chemical dump became undeniable. It was found that the odds for contracting cancer were as high as 1 in 10 for anyone living in a home on the edge of the site, and this calculation took into account only chemicals in the air, neglecting the known contamination in the soil and underground water table. Love Canal was one environmental time bomb that went off.

Perhaps the most underrated and misunderstood environmental pollutant is noise, which usually is regarded more as a nuisance than as a health menace. While most people recognize that impairment of hearing is a danger, few realize that forty epidemiological studies in eleven nations have all linked excessive noise exposure to cardiovascular disorders. The measurable reactions include decrease in gastric juices, increased intracranial pressure, constriction of muscles, skin reactions, the release of adrenal hormones, and increased blood pressure. Exposure to high noise levels can be an immediate danger to those suffering from circulatory diseases, heart problems, and high blood pressure, and it inflicts long-term wear and tear on everyone.

The unit used to measure noise is the decibel, 1 decibel being the lowest sound that can be heard by a human ear under quiet conditions. The measurement indicates the amount of pressure on the ear, and the numbers rise logarithmically, so that an increase from 0 decibels to 120 is an increase of 10 to the twelfth power. Serious health effects commence at about 80 decibels, and at 140 decibels there is pain. A whisper is about 20 decibels, a ticking watch 30, a vacuum cleaner 75, heavy traffic 80, a motorcycle 95, a subway car 105, amplified music 110, and a large jet engine 125 at a distance of 75 feet. A home in the country will usually be in the 20–30 decibel range, while an apartment in New York will be in the 50–70 range, depending on the time of day and district. Factories are usually in the danger area, with considerable variation from department to department.

Just as spicy foods have to become increasingly spicier to be tasted because taste buds are destroyed, loud noises beget louder noises as the ear's ability to hear deteriorates. The contemporary fad for highly amplified music and delight in loud noises feeds upon itself and upon the hearing difficulties of workers who do not protect their hearing at work with earplugs and other devices. Booming discotheque loudspeakers put out from 115 to 130 decibels, while a riveter's gun heard at thirty feet is over 110 decibels.

In terms of life extension, the major danger from noise is the long-term wear and tear it does as a stressor. Hearing tests given at high schools and colleges revealed that hearing is deteriorating much sooner than in previous generations. To avoid the rapid aging that is associated with such a syndrome, the would-be longevous will want to bypass any occupation in which unavoidable noise levels greater than 80 decibels are a condition of work, and they will arrange their living in a manner in which noise is under control. Political activism at a local level can play a significant role in noise abatement. The difference in cost between a loud garbage truck or subway car and quiet ones is negligible and a sum saved many times over in medical expenses and human dignity.

Anyone with a shred of social consciousness or any thought for posterity must be concerned with environmental pollution. But for strictly selfish reasons, the need for action is even more urgent. As the twentieth century moves to a close, environmental pollution is emerging as a major threat to long life and health everywhere in the world. Cancer, which is already the number two killer in the United States and on the increase, is bound intimately with pollution, whether the form be particulate matter, radiation, petrochemicals, or toxins. These same pollutants play an additional negative role in heart disease, which is the number one killer; in many respiratory diseases; in birth defects; and in other threats to life. Since terracidal technologies and chemistries are not essential for human survival, playing Russian roulette with talk of environmental "trade-offs" and "acceptable risks" is unjustified. It amounts to no more than an excuse for a monstrous greed that values short-term private profit at the cost of long-term threats to all life forms.

Individual responses can reduce many environmental dangers by 50 to 80 percent, but these threats need not exist at all, and there is the ever-present danger of falling victim to some unsuspected source. The only acceptable permanent solution is general detoxification of society through control of pollution at its source. Achieving such an end will be as arduous a struggle as that experienced by the nineteenth-century sanitation reformers whose efforts culminated in a near doubling of the average life-span. The same combination of governmental timidity, private avarice, and professional arrogance is once again in opposition to structural change. It is to be hoped that the required political mandate for genuine progress will be mustered without the need to suffer a planetary cancer epidemic or a global acidic rain.

13

REDEFINING
THE BIOLOGICAL LIMITS

> This problem [aging] should be
> solved with even more resolution
> than that devoted to the solving of
> the A-bomb problem a while back,
> or the current problem of conquer-
> ing the cosmos.
>
> —*L. V. Komarov*

During the Age of Enlightenment, European scientists began
to think of the universe as being like a clock. A creator had
fashioned the parts, wound them up, and set the mechanism
working according to fixed laws, which humans eventually
could master for the betterment of their lives. By the
twentieth century the clock metaphor had been extended to
the interior of the human body, which often was described as
containing numerous individual systemic clocks. Proper
nutrition, exercise, and medical treatment would keep the
clocks working efficiently. It also was possible to speculate
that the clocks could be rewound periodically, perhaps a
limited number of times, perhaps infinitely. Almost without
notice the ancient dream of rejuvenation and immortality
had passed from the imaginative realm of myth into the
rational methodology of the research laboratory.[1]

Any rewinding of biological clocks entails the development of a unified theory of aging. Strangely enough, even though aging occurs in all times and places, proceeding through the various parts of the human organism at a fairly predictable speed, there is no satisfactory explanation as to why aging happens or how it is regulated. Treatment for aging must address symptoms rather than causes. But if the causes of aging could be determined, aging would be reduced to the category of a disease. The prospect would then be to modify the effects of or totally eliminate causes of aging: the ultimate cure for the ultimate disease.

This staggering vision is no longer limited to science-fiction writers. The work done in microbiology since the 1930s has been as revolutionary as that seen in physics during the earlier decades of the century. Just as theoretical physics was to culminate in the birth of the nuclear age by mid-century, by the end of the century the new biology is expected to make a revolutionary impact on aging. Even before a breakthrough that might put all previous limits on the human life-span up for redefinition, it is likely that there will be a series of advances, each of which could add five, ten, or twenty years to the average life-span. The implications for persons who will be no more than 80 years of age by A.D. 2000 are unprecedented. Instead of their being at the cusp of old age, their projected life-spans may be extendable by decades, with the accelerating possibility of living to enjoy new advances that make additional extensions possible.

A detailed evaluation of the scientific principles and rudimentary experiments pioneered by antiaging specialists is beyond the scope of this book. More relevant is what changes in life-style could be safely adopted in view of the preliminary findings and what insights that work offers into the longevity components already identified. Having a basic orientation to antiaging research also puts an individual on guard against adopting reckless measures that may be recommended on the basis of incomplete or misunderstood experimental research. The disposition toward fraud and wishful thinking in rejuvenation products and techniques exceeds even that of centenarian age claims.

The simplest hypothesis on aging is that there is a mechanism within the body, perhaps in the brain, hypothalamus, or pituitary, which releases an enzyme, a hormone, a substance *x* which signals the body to start closing down its systems. The discovery of such a mechanism, if it indeed exists, would make it possible to devise a counteraging magic bullet which would keep the substance from being released, delay its release, hamper its effectiveness, or destroy it.

Similar to the death-substance theory is the idea that aging results from coding in the basic DNA or in errors made through the linking RNA of each cell. The error phenomenon has been compared to a duplicating machine in which subsequent copies or copies made from copies are never quite as clear as the original. Eventually the dot to an *i* gets left off or a *t* is left uncrossed or a message is smudged. It is observable that as cells age, their errors multiply. Consequently, as cells are replaced through division, errors accumulate more rapidly. Part of the problem may stem from outside factors like radiation which destroy part of the DNA and RNA, but structural problems in the genetic instructions cannot be ruled out.

Whatever the source of cellular error, should genetic engineering or genetic surgery ever become a reality, a physician would be able to readjust the DNA and RNA to their original efficiency. It also might be possible to take disease-fighting cells from a person during his or her early teens when those cells are extremely vigorous, freeze them, and then reintroduce them into the body at a later time when the cells left in the body have become weaker and less efficient. Ultimately the genetic code itself may be alterable. When this is possible, diseases based on genetic inheritance would become curable.

Another aspect of cellular error under intensive investigation is the immunological system of the body. As the organism ages, the white blood cells find it harder to distinguish between dangerous or unhealthy cells and cells that are sound. New cells sometimes are treated as hostile microbes. The body, in effect, begins to attack itself. No one has been able to understand why this occurs or how it may be prevented. Autoimmunity may be linked to the presence of a general death agent, accumulated cellular errors, or as yet unknown factors. There is some hope that hormones might be able to combat this phenomenon. For example, thymosin, a hormone produced by the thymus gland, has been found effective in the treatment of some autoimmune conditions.

Cross linkage of protein molecules is yet another of the cellular-aging theories. The term refers to the hardening of connective tissues and has been likened to cells that are glued together or toughened in the way leather is in tanning. The hardened connective tissue becomes less able to deliver oxygen, nutrients, hormones, and other substances to the cells. It is suspected that some soil-bacteria enzymes might break down cross linkage. Thus, soil analysis of any area where there seems to be unusual longevity has become standard. Although no enzyme or other substance has yet been found to combat cross linkage, tobacco smoking and radiation are known to encourage it.

In addition to cross linkage, cellular interactions produce unneeded by-products sometimes referred to as intercellular sludge, cellular garbage, and clinkers. While it is not clear whether these should be thought of as causes or products of aging, they cause considerable damage. Viewed as a group, clinkers may be seen as so much corrosion or dust interfering with the delicate settings of the internal biological clocks. Various combinations of vitamins and antioxidants in combination with low-fat diets are being investigated to determine which would be most effective in preventing the accumulation of the garbage in the first place, in escorting the debris out of the body, or in chemically transforming it into more useful compounds. Practical recommendations for the diet or supplements to the diet should be forthcoming before the end of the century.

A more fundamental role for the cell in aging is proposed by Dr. Leonard Hayflick. In the late 1950s, Hayflick created a biological revolution when he overturned the view that the individual human cell is immortal. His experiments showed that with the intriguing exception of cancerous cells, each human cell grown in culture is limited to fifty (plus or minus ten) reproductions or doublings. If this limit applies to cells growing in the body as well, the cellular life-span of humans would be between one hundred and one hundred and twenty years. It also opens the possibility of nuclear cellular transplants for purposes of life extension rather than simple disease fighting. Cells that had gone through only some of their potential divisions could be taken from an individual and kept in cold storage. At a later date, the cells would be returned to the donor to complete their pairings. Although there would be a finite limit to the body, its life would be considerably longer than the wildest supercentenarian claim. The exact methodology required would be formidable, to say the least, but as the cells of even the most elderly people have some doublings left, Hayflick's work provides evidence from yet another perspective that no one has ever died of old age. Furthermore, his work has triggered speculation that cell divisions might be extended through various chemical interventions. One experiment using Vitamin E appears to have increased doublings to over one hundred, or twice the Hayflick limit.

Another intervention proposed at the cellular level is chemical tampering with the bodily temperature. It is estimated that if the body's thermostat could be lowered by from 2 to 3 degrees Celsius, there would be no negative side effects, while life might be extended from twenty to thirty years. This lowering could be accomplished through drugs, genetic engineering, mechanical devices, or mind techniques. One proposal involves a sleeping device or chamber which could lower the temperature of the body at rest to near freezing in the manner of a hibernating bear—a perspective with echoes of the Soviet observation that the long-living people of the Caucasus live under slightly refrigerated circumstances.

Looking forward a few centuries to the age of intergalactic travel, suspended animation through freezing could overcome the problem of voyages that might last a hundred or more earth years. Part of the crew could be kept alive but frozen for months or years at a time. The conscious lifetime would not be increased, but the overall lifetime would be spread out over an incredible period. One hundred crew members on a hundred-year voyage might each be awake for only ten years. If no one was over 35 at the time of lift-off, no one would be more than 45 on landing, even though a hundred years had elapsed.

A contemporary attempt to gain entry into the super-longevous future through freezing is called cryonics. This method involves the placing of a fresh corpse in a container and freezing it to the temperature of liquid nitrogen. Its advocates hope that the process will preserve the body in a state of suspended animation until such time as the diseases that killed the body can be reversed or until aging itself has become a curable disease. The problems associated with cryonics are enormous. Even its most optimistic supporters acknowledge that the present freezing technology may be so primitive that the chance of successful revival is exceedingly slim, a mere percentage of 1 percent. A problem less candidly addressed is that the body should not be dead at the time of freezing if positive results are to be anticipated; yet if the body is not technically dead, then the freezing itself might be legally definable as murder. Because of this dilemma, secrecy surrounds any cryonic encapsulation. As of 1980, it was estimated that 34 bodies had been frozen and that 80 other persons had made arrangements for encapsulation at death. Although some bodies had to be prematurely thawed because the financial arrangements made before death went awry, insurance policies were available that would guarantee the maintenance of the cryonic chamber for hundreds of years.

The cryonics movement is championed by extremely articulate spokespeople who say that however slim the chance of revival, it is better than no chance at all. Just what "slim" means is indicated by an experiment done in the late 1970s at Berkeley. A healthy dog had its blood flushed out and replaced with chemicals which reduced its temperature to below freezing. After the animal had been in frozen suspended animation for one-half hour, the chemicals were flushed out and the blood restored. The dog regained consciousness but survived only seventeen hours before expiring for good. Such episodes suggest that like those ancient Egyptians who placed their faith in mummification, the cryonicists, rather than becoming the first immortalists, are more likely to be museum curios of the future.

In opposition to the theories which place the major cause of aging within the organism itself are theories of wear and tear, which hold that the body is aged, for the most part, by relentless outside pressures. These hostile forces include emotional factors, physical collisions, and environmental pollutants of every description. A bridge between this view and the autoimmunologic theory is that any force which weakens the body from the outside may so disorient the immunological defense system that it begins to make errors. The process accelerates as more and more irreplaceable cells are lost, and the body's slowing ability to recover makes stresses such as noise progressively more annoying. In *Prolongevity*,[2] the most readable and most comprehensive popular work on antiaging research, Albert Rosenfeld points out that almost every facet of aging eventually is connected to all others and can be used to explain them. Until there is a unified law of aging, it will be difficult to separate some effects from some causes or to put aging factors into a hierarchical order of menace.

Rosenfeld is sympathetic to the view that the organism may face a multiplicity of agers. Perhaps there is a substance which signals the body to slow down, but if it should fail in its mission, there are backup systems. The limitation of cell doublings or autoimmunological errors or cross linkage or cellular garbage will slow down the organism, and if they do not, never-ending wear and tear will. A more optimistic view is that bodily programs are aimed at survival of the species, with death an irrelevant consideration. This view emphasizes that the body is coded to have its major systems in prime condition during the reproductive stage of life. What happens afterward may not be genetically programmed. Alex Comfort has used the analogy of a spacecraft designed to photograph Mars on a bypass flight. All the craft's systems will be in top operational efficiency during the most advantageous periods for taking pictures, and there will be no energy wasted on self-destruct systems. The craft may be unlucky and collide with an object in the asteroid belt. Some of its parts may fail or be damaged by cosmic rays. Or it may be trapped by the gravitational field of a planet, either becoming an artificial moon or being pulled into the atmosphere until it is consumed like a falling star. The craft might, however, escape the Solar System altogether and become an intergalactic voyager. The implications for humans are that if the body is not programmed to self-destruct, the medical problem for life extension is immensely simplified. Rather than thwarting coded death systems, the prolongevous physician will be concerned with maintenance and repair problems.

Thinking of the body as a machine requiring maintenance leads to the need for replacing as well as repairing worn-out parts. Automobile life may be extended for decades, but only if components are replaced as part of the general upkeep. The wooden peg leg and iron arm hook were among the first human spare parts to be widely used. Today science has provided pacemakers for tired hearts, plastic tubing for destroyed arteries, mechanical joints for worn-out bones, and transplants for dysfunctioning organs. Perhaps some future philosophers will be debating at what point an organism contains so many artificial parts that it ceases to be human and should be thought of as an android or robot. Long before that hypothetical era, however, bionic spare parts and other techniques will be making a substantial impact on comfort in old age and on life extension. Cameralike devices and miniaturized radio technology already have raised the possibility that afflictions like blindness and deafness may become as obsolete as smallpox.

A more spectacular technique mentioned in relation to providing human spare parts is cloning. To judge from procedures now possible with simple life forms, scientists may at some future time be able to use a cell from a human donor to construct a body that would be an identical twin. Futurist writers have projected the possibility of having a spare clone body for each human, which could serve as an ideal organ bank, since the identical genetic codes would eliminate problems of tissue rejection. The ultimate in this line of reasoning is that a clone could be created and kept in suspended animation without activation of the brain. When the donor's original body began to fail, the donor's memory bank could be transferred to the clone: a de facto self-rebirth. That such a scenario could ever become possible is problematical. The subject is worthy of mention only to indicate the fantastic projections that are now theoretically consistent with established scientific canon. The fact that they appear to be possible does not guarantee that they actually are or that if possible, they are necessarily desirable.

Contrasting with superscience methods such as cloning or bionic parts is antiaging research that draws from traditional lore. As the physical effects of stress have become recognized as potent antilongevous factors, there has been a resurgence of interest in ways of reducing stress damage through techniques that promote the mental mobilization of internal bodily energy. Methods rooted in the ancient practice of yoga have been measured objectively and have been found capable of lowering the pressure of the blood, slowing the beating of the heart, reducing the tension in muscles, and improving the amount of oxygen in the blood. Similar benefits have been obtained by people working with biofeedback, methods by which individuals use electronic devices and graphs to listen to their own vital signs in order to regulate them through purely mental techniques.

Although listening to one's brain waves is just a game to many people and meditation exercises often have associated mystical overloads, the use of the mind to monitor bodily responses without recourse to medical or surgical intervention would be an invaluable contribution to fighting off premature aging. The biggest drawback to this kind of research moving along scientific lines is that individuals of the kind attracted to biofeedback and meditation often wish to minimize the role of exercise, diet, and life-style in reducing the premature aging being addressed. Moreover, it is unlikely that mind control could ever check the destructive effect of a force like radiation or a large dose of arsenic. Rather than a single answer to aging, mind techniques are additional or alternative weapons in the prolongevity arsenal aimed at preventing or alleviating the wear-and-tear damage of stress.

Another antiaging front rooted in traditional knowledge is the search for a perfect food. Robert Prehoda has written of a future when there will be a synthetic food that improves upon the chemistry of Mother Nature by providing the optimal bodily fuel in a form that causes the least amount of internal wear and tear.[3] Today's health tonics, multivitamin supplements, and hormonal injections are the initial steps in this direction, and finding the most effective antioxidants and determining the exact role of various hormones, enzymes, minerals, and vitamins remains the present focus of antiaging dietary research. Progress must necessarily be slow, as many food elements have the double edge to them already described in relation to mineral supplements. Long-term observation of human volunteers, possible only after long-term experiments with other mammals, will be needed before a better general diet of conventional foods can be authoritatively drawn. Minimum daily requirements for many nutrients have not been established, and levels for most are in dispute.

Before a single synthetic food or dietary regimen is available for tailoring to biochemical individuality, there will be a series of modest improvements in nutrition which will steadily upgrade the diet. But this process cannot be forced. The life-extension claims that have been made for some antioxidants, tranquilizers, and metals are strictly premature, having no verifiable base. To put them into the body on a regular basis is to play the guinea pig for posterity, a role that may be honorable but one not to be taken lightly or under false illusions as to the risk involved. Prolongevous optimists must realize that when an experiment is called "promising" the adjective is not a blanket go-ahead signal so much as a warning that the findings are tentative. Unsuspected side effects, such as those associated with prolonged estrogen therapy, may develop, or the procedure may prove to have only a passing effect. Claims rooted in Soviet research must be judged against the repeated announcements by Dimitri Chebotarev, the dean of Soviet aging research, that even the most positive Soviet findings remain strictly experimental and that the procedures and substances so far developed should not be used in general treatment but limited to well-monitored research projects.

The historical precedents for ignoring cautionary advice such as that of Chebotarev are not very encouraging. Typical is the turn-of-the-century attempt of older men to become sexually rejuvenated through grafts or injections derived from the testicles of goats and monkeys. Except for psychological support, the procedures simply didn't work. What might have been just another amusing example of human gullibility became tragic when one set of grafts inadvertently used syphilitic monkeys, transferring that disease to the humans at a time when penicillin had not yet been discovered.[4]

Sexual rejuvenation also figures heavily in a rejuvenation technique favored by the wealthy and available for decades—cell transplants from lambs. Developed by Dr. Paul Niehans, the method is based on the assumption that liver cells will rejuvenate the liver, heart cells the heart, kidney cells the kidney, and so forth. Treatment at Niehans' lush Swiss clinic became popular among the elite of Europe during the 1930s, and his claims got a tremendous boost when cell transplants to Pope Pius XII were followed by that pontiff's recovery from a serious illness which had resisted previous treatments. Although most of Niehans' patients prefer to remain anonymous, a few, including Somerset Maugham, wrote glowingly of the effects of the cell therapy. Generally, however, Niehans has been viewed as part of the beauty-doctor clique rather than as an antiaging scientist. He never published a list of patients who enjoyed unusual life-spans or vigor, and he never published a scientific treatise explaining the how and why of his method. His critics note that Niehans never undertook his own therapy and that when he died, in his late 80s, the signs of his enormous wealth were more visible than any signs of rejuvenation. A number of nations, the United States among them, ban the cell transplants on the grounds that they are useless and perhaps dangerous.

A totally different antiaging arena attempts to determine what health effects result from climatic forces such as cosmic rays, barometric pressure, electromagnetism, and sunspot activity. Investigators have found that bodily temperatures adjust to diurnal rhythms, falling in the evening and rising in the earlier part of the day. One of the causes of the phenomenon known as "jet lag" is that when a body has moved rapidly through time zones or from northern to southern hemisphere, its physical responses are no longer synchronized with the new pattern of night and day or summer and winter. The greater the distance traveled, the greater the likelihood of a period of disorientation and readjustment. Positive correlations also have been found between outbreaks of lymphocytosis and increases in solar activity; and some weather fronts seem to be accompanied by an increase in the number of hospital admissions. It is not clear whether the fronts or solar outbursts trigger a crisis about to occur in any case or whether they are causes of the ailment. Nor is it certain that the correlations so far uncovered would hold up under a longer, more comprehensive time period. Related work has attempted to determine the cause-and-effect relationship between prevailing winds in Europe and diseases that come in their wake. If definite connections were established, it might be possible to give warning forecasts such as those issued when the air quality is dangerous. Individuals found to have higher sensitivity to certain types of weather could adjust their behavior for heightened or lessened efficiency.[5]

Soviet researchers have been looking at the longevous effects of positive and negative air ions. Their work has included field studies in the areas of the Caucasus with the highest centenarian concentrations, but remains inconclusive. Scientists in other countries have used negative air ions in the successful treatment of third-degree burns. Once the benefits and dangers of positive and negative air ions have been comprehensively catalogued, it may be possible to regulate ionization in enclosures such as homes and offices. In addition, serious attention could be given to using natural or synthetic fabrics that most effectively mediate between climatic forces and bodily reactions.

Promising as these many facets of antiaging research are, the work is severely handicapped by inadequate funding. If the United States ever decided to invest in a Methuselah Project in the way it once invested in the Manhattan Project to develop a nuclear bomb, a series of significant breakthroughs could be achieved rather speedily. But this is not likely to occur. The achievement of extended life-spans stirs fears about the social and economic readjustments that would be required in a society where there would be considerable numbers of people over 80. A whole body of writing has already come into being to address such questions theoretically, but most government-connected scientists and social planners are greatly troubled by the prospect. Another spectrum of opposition stems from those whose religious orientation makes them uneasy about genetic tampering and even such relatively simple medical interventions as contraception, artificial insemination and abortion. Among the great powers, the Soviet Union has given the most support to longevity scientists, but when compared with its outlays for military projects, the amounts spent are inconsiderable. In nations less self-sufficient than the U.S.A. and the U.S.S.R., problems of inadequate national resources and technological underdevelopment make population reduction or stabilization a higher national priority than antiaging research. The bulk of research, as a result, remains underfinanced and uncoordinated.

The only major area in which the primary interests of the great powers intersect with longevity research is space exploration. As plans for manned space platforms, moon colonies, and interplanetary travel move toward realization, the search for optimal foods, fabrics, exercises, atmospheres, and the like ceases to be utopian and becomes pragmatic. The whole adventure of humans in space also presents the first opportunity to observe reactions of the body to various cosmic influences when it is not surrounded by a protective atmosphere developed over the millennia.

In the long run, the brunt of antiaging research remains in the domain of medicine proper. One can say that all medical research is a fight to extend life and delay death. Although, ultimately, every doctor loses every patient, medicine continues to deny that failure, at any given moment, is necessary. Every small medical advance hastens the day when life-spans will approach the genetic limits. At the same time, work such as recombinant DNA research, at once the most dangerous and the most revolutionary biology ever conceived, questions whether any genetic program should be considered a final arbiter of age.

The scenario for successful antiaging progress in the last decades of the twentieth century is that even before the elaboration of a unified law of aging, incremental gains in knowledge will steadily redefine the quality and duration of life. Encouraging as this prospect is, the average person must always differentiate between methods which seek to aid us in reaching the present genetic limits and those which defy those and all other limits. The acceptance strategy aims to make individual behavior more harmonious with forces that have been interacting in a predictable fashion for as long as humans have observed them. The defiance strategy, on the other hand, would remake the rules of the cosmic game, creating situations for which precedents may be irrelevant. Doomsday chemicals or cellular tampering that would make present life-spans appear like a paradise lost are just as possible as a future in which life is calculated in centuries rather than years. The stakes are so awesome and the ground so uncertain that societies, like individuals, had best proceed with extreme caution. The years of Methuselah and even physical immortality may be waiting somewhere along the time—space continuum, but they are not around the gerontological corner. And there is no assurance that science fictions will become scientific realities.

14

LONGEVITY NOW

Long Life to You

Never before in the history of the human race has choice rather than chance played the dominant role in how long any given person shall live. Particularly in developed nations, there has been a greatly lowered risk of bodily injuries due to inadequate food supplies, serious infectious disease, and the need to work to the point of exhaustion. At the same historical juncture, the activities, diet, and attitudes most conducive to long life have begun to emerge from the haze of anecdotal folklore to become objectively verifiable. It is useful, therefore, to reexamine the essentials of the longevity agenda to see just what the major prolongevous decisions are and how they affect the statistical prospects for long life.

Until such time as genetic manipulation becomes a reality, the outer limits of any individual's life will be determined by his or her genetic code. Examining all of the best claims available shows that there is no case of a documented life-span reaching 115 years. Assuming that among the much larger undocumented population there may be some persons who have lived longer, the outer limit of life under the most favorable conditions could be extended to no more than one hundred and twenty years. More practically, even among centenarians, already a statistical fraction, few will survive after 105 and almost none after 110. What, then, are the real chances that any given American will live to enjoy a 100th birthday?

The answer is complicated by the difficulty of establishing the exact number of living centenarians. The most optimistic U.S. figures are found in raw census data, which reported 4,447 centenarians in 1950, 10,369 centenarians in 1960, and 106,441 centenarians in 1970. The problem with these figures is that they are based on the simple assertions of those interviewed or on the assertions of relatives or friends. As in other nations, the number of reported centenarians in the United States is highest where illiteracy is highest, and investigations of specific claims show that if there is any tendency to falsification it is to lie upward. Although the census takers might miss a few individuals, particularly those living in remote rural areas where the number of centenarians might be highest, the exaggerations would more than make up for the omissions.

Statisticians have always been leery of centenarian data based on census returns and have devised means for testing their validity.[1] Jacob Siegel and Jeffrey Passel, demographic statisticians in the population division of the U.S. Bureau of the Census, have examined the centenarian data of 1950, 1960, and 1970 and have concluded that the counts are off by as much as 95 percent.[2] This evaluation is based on three independent verification procedures. The simplest involves a comparison of current Medicare data with census material. More complex are calculations called the Forward Survival Method and the Population Reconstruction Method. Each of the procedures is worthy of separate consideration.

All Americans over the age of 65 became eligible for

various benefits under the Social Security System in 1965. This was a departure from the previous practice of requiring that a person had to have paid into the system in order to receive any benefits. By 1970 the number of centenarians enrolled under Medicare was a little over 7,000—a far cry from the 106,441 centenarians reported in the census of that same year. It could be argued that many centenarians were psychologically unprepared to accept government assistance, didn't need it, or were ignorant of their eligibility. The disparity, however, is too mammoth for such a view to be entertained seriously. It is more likely that since Medicare requires some proof of age, the octogenarians and non-agenarians who had lied to the census taker reported their true ages to Social Security. The number could still be inflated, as Social Security is not particularly interested in how old a person is as long as he or she is over 65. The case of Charlie Smith comes to mind. Again, if there were any tendency to falsification, it would be to lie upward in order to take benefits sooner. This would mean that persons who had lied upward at around age 50 or 60 eventually would be pushed into the centenarian ranks prematurely. The Social Security records will be much more dependable in the first decades of the new century when those who entered the system (founded in 1935) in their youth and who can be traced continuously start to become centenarians. Even before that time, the Social Security statistics are probably more accurate in counting older people than the census is.

The Forward Survival Method of determining cente-narians correlates the centenarians of 1970 with the number of nonagenarians in 1960 and the number of octogenarians in 1950. Applying the mortality rates for nonagenarians and octogenarians during that time, it is possible to determine how many of the octogenarians of 1950 were nonagenarians in 1960 and how many of those nonagenarians became centenarians in 1970. Obviously, unless there had been a flood of nonagenarian immigrants during the 1960s, there couldn't possibly be more centenarians in 1970 than there were nonagenarians in 1960. Using figures from 1959 through 1961, Siegel and Passel found that in 1970 there would be 3,395 centenarians. Working in some of the Medicare figures, they came up with 7,113, but by including figures from 1949 through 1951, they reduced the number to 3,222.

Siegel and Passel also employed the Population Reconstruction Method, which starts with a group of 100,000 infants and, using different methods of determining mortality rates, follows the group, called a cohort, until all of its members are deceased. Using one set of variations the team came up with 8,211 centenarians for 1970 and using another arrived at a figure of 7,854. Both of these were slightly higher than the Medicare numbers but, again, were dwarfed by those of the census.

The drawbacks to both the Forward Survival and Population Reconstruction approaches is that they are influenced by the same census data in question and involve abstract mathematical formulations not always consistent with changing reality. It is possible, for example, that the death rates which follow a predictable curve through the tenth decade change thereafter because they are freed from the distortions of premature aging, and it is possible that the slow accumulation of health increments is changing the ratios that have been valid previous to 1970. Taking some of these doubts into consideration and comparing their various findings, Siegel and Passel believe that the actual number of centenarians in 1970 was about 4,800. Most life-insurance experts and other statisticians interested in the subject of centenarians concur with this figure. Relating the American data to centenarian counts in other developed nations, it is generally agreed that out of every 100,000 persons born in the United States, 3 to 5 will live to be at least 100 years of age, with women having a 2-to-1 advantage over men.

On first consideration, the centenarian counts appear to be pretty disheartening for those who would be longevous. But using other statistics of equal merit, a much more optimistic vista is obtained. From 1960 to 1980 the population of the United States got progressively older, a tendency expected to continue until at least the turn of the twenty-first century. One of the characteristics of the aging American was that he or she was getting increasingly healthier. This could be seen in the finding that the percentage as well as the number of people at all age levels over 60 was growing steadily. The average age at which individuals entered nursing homes during the 1970s rose from 76 to 82, with the average age at death in those homes climbing accordingly. This improvement in statistical averages is particularly significant for those adhering to prolongevous life-styles, because the death rates at all ages continued to be highest for those who smoke, overeat, are inactive, use many petrochemicals, are overradiated, and otherwise expose their bodies to established death risks. In this respect, the golden lining of the longevity agenda is that it is not an all-or-nothing proposition. While close adherence will substantially increase the possibility of reaching 100, even reasonable adherence will definitely increase the odds for a robust 70 or 80—odds which already are about 2 to 1 at the end of the first year of life and which get progressively better with each additional year of survival.

More support for prolongevous life-styles is found by examination of the leading causes of death. Major newspapers in early 1980 reported that Dr. Donald Millar, assistant director of the National Center for Disease Control, had stated that the stunning increase in the national average life-span was not likely to continue because the major causes of mortality were due to poor individual and societal choices which showed few signs of positive change.[3] The rise in the overall consumption of alcohol and the continued high level of smoking were two examples cited. Millar estimated that about 50 percent of the mortality in the United States was due to unhealthful behavior or life-style and that another 20 percent was due to environmental factors. This left only 30 percent—20 percent due to biological factors and 10 percent to inadequate health care. This kind of analysis indicates that an individual on a longevity agenda can expect to do much better than the national averages. Much better in this case is nothing less than living longer and healthier.

The longevity agenda that has been developed throughout this book has been based not on the theories or hopes of those who would like to live to be 100, but on the practices of those who have actually done so. Supportive material has been assembled from the lives of tens of thousands of persons who have outperformed the averages. Consequently, as we turn to a final summation, it must be emphasized that if the agenda is to meet any of its four goals, each of the components must be fulfilled according to the standards indicated. While there is considerable room for individual adaptations, any tampering with the basic principles or substitutions based on purely theoretical considerations or isolated experiments is opening the door to wishful thinking.

The component of the longevity agenda least understood by the average person is exercise. There is a decided tendency to seek results obtainable only or most easily through physical activity by some other means. Even individuals who do become convinced of its central importance often cling to sports or other routines which they happen to enjoy or to which they are accustomed regardless of whether they are truly prolongevous in nature. Many people find it hard to accept that one of the best ways to prevent premature aging is the simple act of walking. If the amount of vigorous lifelong physical activity recommended as optimal appears somewhat unusual, it is well to remember that it is unusual for people to live to be 100, or even 90.

Far more popular than exercise is concern for diet. This method of influencing health is actually too popular, for many people would have it substitute for all other longevity factors. As a result, many unusual eating habits are considered essential to long life by persons otherwise possessed of common sense. At the other extreme are people who knowingly eat poorly because of ceremonial, social, occupational, or psychological pressures. It is a rare person who consistently has the fortitude to think of food as fuel for the body and who insists on having the best fuel available.

Two methods used to determine the best bodily fuels are analysis of the digestive system and examination of the diets of longevous people. Both procedures yield a diet that is predominantly or exclusively vegetarian, consisting of as many raw foods and as wide a variety of foods as possible, with freshness and quality of paramount importance. This overall diet is low in fat, sugar, salt, and calories. If followed regularly, it protects the body from a number of degenerative diseases, not the least of which are arterial conditions associated with the accumulation of cellular garbage. Cancer of the breast, the leading cancer killer among American females during the decade of the 1970s, and cancer of the rectum and colon, the second leading cancer killer for both sexes during the same period, are both rare among vegetarians. The combination of a vigorous life-style and prolongevous eating habits should produce a lean somatype. The exact shape and weight of the body will be influenced by genetic factors, but in all events will be much slimmer and probably shorter than that thought of as healthy or pleasing in most cultures. The accumulation of excess weight often begins in infancy with the mistaken parental belief that a fat baby is a healthy baby. Later, there will be pressure on mature men to be more muscular and on mature women to be fatter than is prolongevously desirable. At about the fortieth year of life, when the metabolic rate begins to slow, reduced eating or increased exercise will be necessary to prevent weight accumulation. While it is an error to think correlation automatically means causation, lower body weight correlates negatively with all major diseases and positively with long life.

Although not as easily quantifiable as exercise, dietary, and weight factors, the behavioral component of the longevity agenda is critical. Either by choice or by circumstance, longevous people usually live in situations that nurture them, labor at work they find rewarding, and possess a high degree of self-esteem. Their lives proceed in orderly and rhythmic patterns, with periodic changes dictated by the seasons or changing generational responsibilities. Although extremely active, they are not harried by time pressure and do not work to exhaustion. Formal retirement is uncommon; and self-esteem, which may be wedded to family roles, social commitments, or personal creativity, usually increases with the passage of time. The longevous avoid chronologically defined ghettos and set themselves high levels of expectation. In combination, these personality traits and behavioral patterns decrease the stress damage possible from psychological and physical tension. Historically, many of the longevous have lived in societies in which orderly routines were socially programmed and in which self-image was derived from strictly defined social functions. These conditions do not obtain in advanced technological societies. Inhabitants of such societies must be far more self-directed in ordering daily life and establishing long-term personal and familial goals.

The biographies of the longevous indicate that they have strong ideas about health and have much less contact with physicians than most people. They tend to be somewhat unimpressed with new medications and scientific approaches that have not withstood a reasonable test of time. The longevous seem to tolerate professional medical advice rather than being in awe of it. Few of them have a history of taking nutritional supplements or drugs on a regular basis. A rule that can be formulated from their behavior is that no supplements or medicines should be used before there is a demonstrated need. When treatment of a disease is required, nutritional or physical-therapy cures are the preferred methods of healing. If they are not viable options, a number of opinions should be sought to determine which of the available treatments represents the best chance of recovery with the least assault on normal bodily functions.

A major component of any contemporary longevity agenda is the avoidance of cancer-causing stimuli. An individual can gain considerable protection by avoiding tobacco smoke, by being on guard against industrial pollutants, by rejecting adulterated food, and by limiting his or her exposure to radiation. This personal program should be accompanied by vigorous support for political efforts to detoxify the environment so that air, water, and soil can be returned to the purity of bygone eras. Clever industrial propaganda to the effect that all life is dependent on chemicals and that no chemical is entirely safe in all situations must not obscure the difference between chemicals found in nature and chemicals made in the laboratory. Very few chemicals are carcinogenic, but most that are have been created artificially. How any synthetic product will react when it is let loose in nature is unpredictable. Whenever the safety of a new chemical or a new source of radiation is piously assured, the ten-to-forty-year latency period for cancer should be considered. The fundamental rule is that abnormal stimuli are likely to promote abnormal bodily responses.

After so much human effort has been expended to find some exotic "secret" to long life, it is somewhat ironic that the simplest life-styles and some of the most natural bodily responses are key longevity factors. Rather than extending the life-span or rejuvenating the body, prolongevous habits maintain the body's resistance to premature aging. Someday, it may become possible to reset the internal biological clocks. Until then, the reasonable expectation of life should be from ninety to one hundred and five years. To achieve this goal, the would-be longevous steadfastly refuse to be victimized by human folly and ignorance. They reject a toxic society in which disease is considered normal and insist that it is possible to construct healthy societies in which the mass of humanity will die of old age. Prolongevous planning by individuals and groups is a bold stretching for the biological limits, a demand to live each of the decades for which the body has been programmed and to live each of those decades with zest.

BIBLIOGRAPHIC ESSAY AND NOTES

Given the diverse nature of individual chapters, other materials consulted (but not cited) have been added to the notes for that chapter under the heading Additional Sources. Books and articles on the general subject of longevity are listed with the notes for Chapter 7 ("Rethinking the First Ninety-Nine"). The note entries and additional sources make up a selected bibliography. Full reference information is given each time a source is cited for the first time within any particular chapter.

Notes to Introduction

1. A good rendition of immortality episodes in the Gilgamesh myth and commentary can be found in Theodor H. Gaster, *The Oldest Stories in the World* (Boston: Beacon Press, 1952), pp. 21–51.

2. Gerald J. Gruman, *A History of Ideas About the Prolongation of Life* (Philadelphia: The American Philosophical Society, 1966). Similar material is available in Alex Comfort, *The Process of Ageing* (London: Weidenfeld and Nicolson, 1965).

3. An analysis of the changing causes of death in the United States and appropriate charts may be found in Alexander Leaf, *Youth in Old Age* (New York: McGraw-Hill, 1975), pp. xiii–xviii.

4. Recent speculations on the subject were summarized by Jane E. Brody in "Genetic Explanation Offered for Women's Health Superiority," *The New York Times*, January 29, 1980, p. C1.

5. Herbert A. de Vries, *Report on Jogging and Exercise for Older Adults* (Washington D.C.: U.S. Administration on Aging, HEW, 1968); ———, "Physiological Effects of an Exercise Training Regimen Upon Men Aged 52–88," *Journal of Gerontology*, 25: 325–36, 1970; and for exercise guidelines for those over 60, ———, *Vigor Regained* (Englewood Cliffs, New Jersey: Prentice-Hall, Inc., 1974).

6. This is a slight deviation from the guidelnes set in a 1963 meeting of the World Health Organization convened in Kiev. At that conference 60 to 74 was determined to be late maturity, 75 to 89 to be old, and over 90 to be longevous, with no further breakdown.

Notes to Chapter 1: The Oldest of the Old

1. Information about Grandma Filkins has been provided by A. Ross Eckler, who has interviewed some of her descendants. Her obituary appeared in the *Herkimer Evening Telegram* in an issue that is dated December 4, 1928, but appeared about a week later. A low-key notice on the obituary page of *The New York Times* of December 5, 1928, identified her as the oldest woman in the state.

2. William J. Thoms, *The Longevity of Man* (London: Frederic Norgate, 1879). Earlier edition of 1873 also consulted.

3. The entire autopsy report can be found as an appendix in Thoms, *The Longevity of Man*.

4. Leslie Stephen and Sidney Lee, *The Dictionary of National Biography* (London: Oxford University Press, 1950), vol. X, p. 737.

5. T. E. Young, *On Centenarians* (London: Charles and Edwin Layton, 1899). Later 1905 edition also consulted.

6. *Ibid*, pp. 38–42.

7. Maurice Ernest, *The Longer Life* (London: Adam & Co., 1938). The author Anglicized his name during World War I, and some of his work may be found under Ernst.

8. *Ibid.*, p. 37.

9. *Ibid.*, p. 39.

10. *Ibid.*, p. 33.

11. Obituary of Li Chung Yun, *The New York Times*, May 6, 1933, p. 13.

12. Renewed popular interest in ginseng in the 1970s led to more laboratory analysis of the plant in the United States and the Soviet Union. No conclusive results have been forthcoming. However, prolonged use of ginseng has been linked to insomnia, nervousness, diarrhea, and skin eruptions: Ronald K. Siegel, "Ginseng Abuse Syndrome," *Journal of the American Medical Association*, 241:1614–15, 1979. Ironically, Oriental

food faddists of the late 18th and 19th centuries thought American-grown ginseng superior in medicinal powers to that grown elsewhere. This led to a brisk international trade in American-grown ginseng: Leonard Slazinski, Letter and citation in *Journal of the American Medical Association*, 242:616, 1979.

13. The call was placed by Robert Trumbull of the Tokyo Bureau of *The New York Times* after an inquiry from the author. Trumbull also wrote about Izumi in "Japan Hails Elders Amid New Concern for Them," *The New York Times*, September 16, 1979, p. 19. Norman McWhirter, editor of the *Guinness Book of World Records*, provided material independently confirming this data.

14. Rouch did not know of Dollo's possible uniqueness as the oldest person in the world until so informed by the author during an interview dealing with Rouch's films which took place in 1977. The information on Dollo that follows is based on material provided by Rouch at that time and during a follow-up interview a year later by Barbara Margolis.

15. Unsigned article titled "The Man Who Spoke with Lincoln," *Ebony*, February, 1963, pp. 79–84.

16. Obituary for Mark Thrash in *The New York Times*, December 17, 1943, and obituary for Martha Graham in *The New York Times*, June 25, 1959. Additional information from A. Ross Eckler.

17. Zhores Medvedev's major challenge to Soviet data can be found in "Caucasus and Altay Longevity: A Biological or Social Problem?" *The Gerontologist*, October, 1974, vol. 14, no. 5, pp. 381–87, and in "Aging and Longevity," *The Gerontologist*, June, 1975, vol. 15, no. 3, pp. 196–201. A general assessment of Soviet methodology can be found in his *Soviet Science* (New York: Norton, 1978). Medvedev has furnished additional data to the author through a long interview and correspondence.

Notes to Chapter 2:
The Long-Living People of Abkhasia

1. The author had two formal interviews with Dr. Gogoghian in October of 1978 and was able to visit the institute on a number of occasions. Unless otherwise noted, all interviews involving Abkhasians also took place in the first two weeks of October, 1978.

2. G. N. Schinava, N. N. Sachuk, and Sh. D. Gogohiya, "On the Physical Condition of the Aged People of the Abkhasian ASSR," *Soviet Medicine*, 5, 1964, is cited and partly reproduced in Sula Benet, *Abkhasians* (New York: Holt, Rinehart and Winston, 1974), p. 14.

3. *The Guinness Book of World Records* notes: "The oldest recorded mother of whom there is certain evidence is Mrs. Ruth Alice Kistler (née Taylor), formerly Mrs. Shepard, of Portland, Oregon. She was born in Wakefield, Massachusetts, on June 11, 1899, and gave birth to a daughter, Suzan, in Glendale, California, on October 18, 1956, when her age was 57

years, 129 days. Alex Comfort states in *The Process of Ageing* that the oldest recorded father is 94.

4. As of this writing, foreigners may not travel in the U.S.S.R. without preparing and prepaying a day-by-day itinerary, which it is extremely difficult and expensive to alter. The bookings are done through a state agency called Intourist, and the hotel charge in each city includes one official guided tour of the city.

5. Alexander Leaf, *Youth in Old Age* (New York: McGraw-Hill, 1975), p. 8.

6. Sula Benet, *How to Live to Be 100* (New York: Dial Press, 1975), pp. 1–6.

7. Benet, *Abkhasians*, pp. 16–17, 29.

8. Peter Young, "161 Years Old and Going Strong," *Life*, September 16, 1966, vol. 61, no. 12, pp. 121–29.

9. Henry Gris and Milton Merlin, *May You Live to Be 200!* (South Brunswick, N.J., and New York: A. S. Barnes & Co., 1978), pp. 167–84. Gris did all the traveling and research and Merlin handled much of the actual writing.

10. *Ibid.*, p. 172.

11. *Ibid.*, p. 183.

12. Benet, *How . . .*, photographs between pp. 48 and 49.

13. Gris and Merlin, *op. cit.*, p. 273.

14. Mark Bricklin, "Things Here and There," *Prevention*, September, 1978, photograph on p. 82.

15. List of ages provided to the author by Arlene Hoffman, who did the preliminary field research for the Dannon commercials.

16. Alexander Leaf, "Every Day Is a Gift When You Are over 100," *National Geographic*, January, 1973, vol. 143, no. 1, photograph on p. 97.

17. Gris and Merlin, *op. cit.*, pp. 184–206.

18. Benet, *How . . .*, pp. 47–48.

19. *Ibid.*, p. 8.

20. Leaf, *Youth . . .*, p. 20.

21. Gris and Merlin, *op. cit.*, pp. 216–24.

22. Benet, *Abkhasians*, p. 17.

23. Gris and Merlin, *op. cit.*, pp. 225–26.

24. Leaf, "Every Day . . .," p. 104.

25. Gris and Merlin, *op. cit.*, p. 235.

26. John Abercrombey, *A Trip Through the Eastern Caucasus* (London: Edward Standford, 1889), p. 23.

27. Essad Bey, *Twelve Secrets of the Caucasus* (New York: Viking Press, 1931), p. 271.

28. Contemporary Abkhasian writers published include Fazil Eskander, *The Beginning: Short Stories* (Sukhumi: Alashara Press, 1978).

29. Benet, *How . . .*, p. 42.

30. *Ibid.*, p. 43.

31. Elie Metchnikoff, *The Prolongation of Life* (London: William Heinemann, 1910), p. 175.

32. Benet, *How . . .*, p. 48.

33. *Ibid.*, p. 42.

34. Benet, *Abkhasians*, p. 15.

ADDITIONAL SOURCES

Alexander A. Bogomoletz, *The Prolongation of Life* (New York: Duell, Sloan and Pearce, 1946).

Samuel Rosen, Nicolai Preobrajensky, Simeon Khechinashvili, et al., "Epidemiologic Hearing Studies in the U.S.S.R.," *Archives of Otolaryngology*, 1970, vol. 91, no. 5, pp. 424–28.

Notes to Chapter 3: Soviet Centenarians

1. Henry Gris and Milton Merlin, *May You Live to Be 200!* (South Brunswick, N.J., and New York: A. S. Barnes, 1978), p. 143.

2. Dimitry F. Chebotaryov [sic] and Nina N. Sachuk, "Sociomedical Examination of Longevous People in the USSR," *Journal of Gerontology*, October, 1964, vol. 19, no. 4, pp. 435–40; and N. Sachuk, "The Geography of Longevity in the USSR," *Geriatrics*, July, 1965, vol. 20, no. 7, pp. 605–6.

3. Gris and Merlin, *op. cit.*, pp. 278–99, contains a transcript of a taped interview with Chebotarev which contains in one place ideas and observations that can also be found in numerous writings and other interviews.

4. Chebotaryov and Sachuk, "Sociomedical Examination," pp. 435–40; Sula Benet, *How to Live to Be 100* (New York: Dial Press, 1976), p. 52.

5. After an examination of life tables from a variety of statistical statements, L. I. Dublin, A. J. Lotka, and M. Spiegelman, *Length of Life* (New York: Ronald Press Co., 1949) on p. 117 conclude, "These studies indicate that the difference in expectation of life at about age 25 between persons with a better record of parental longevity and those with a poor record may be anywhere between two to four years."

6. Dorothy Gallagher, *Hannah's Daughters* (New York: Thomas Y. Crowell, 1976), genealogy on p. 280, photos on pp. 332 and 333, and Hannah's life story on pp. 13–102.

7. Alexander Graham Bell, "Who Shall Inherit Long Life?" *National Geographic Magazine*, volume XXXV, no. 6, June, 1919, pp. 504–14.

8. Sula Benet, *Abkhasians* (New York: Holt, Rinehart and Winston, 1974), p. 79. Pitskelauri states that 90 percent of Georgian women marry and bear children before age 25 in Patrick M. McGrady, Jr., *The Youth Doctors* (New York: Coward McCann, Inc., 1968), p. 295.

9. Benet, *How . . .*, pp. 145–46.

10. Author's interviews with Peter Lubalin and Arlene Hoffman, summer of 1978.

11. Benet, *op. cit.*, p. 59. Also, the most offspring mentioned for supercentenarians are great grandchildren for a man of 132 in N. Varina (translator), "Secrets of the Centenarians" excerpt from *Literaturnaya Gazeta*, publication of the Soviet Writers' Union in *Atlas World Press Review*, vol. 25, no. 1, January, 1978, p. 46.

12. Benet, *op. cit.*, pp. 55–56.

13. *Ibid.*, p. 58, reported by L. F. Kovalenko of the Institute of Gerontology.

14. Christopher Wren, "Soviet Centenarians," *The New York Times*, September 9, 1977.

15. Gris and Merlin, *op. cit.*, p. 145.

16. Benet, *How . . .*, p. 43. In the final chapter of this book, the correction found most plausible for the raw U.S. census data on centenarians is 95 percent.

17. Gris and Merlin, *op. cit.*, pp. 278–302, 323–26. Also, Dan Fisher, "Soviets Aiming for Lifespan of 400 Years," *Los Angeles Times*, August 13, 1977, p. 1.

18. Gris and Merlin, *op. cit.*, pp. 321–23.

19. Zhores Medvedev, *Soviet Science* (New York: W. W. Norton, 1978), p. 65.

20. Extensive advertising campaign of 1979 in New York City area.

21. Walter C. McKain, "Are They Really That Old?" *The Gerontologist*, 1967, vol. 7, pp. 70–80, and McKain, "The Zone of Health," *The Gerontologist*, 1969, vol. 9, no. 1, pp. 47–54. For a more popular approach: Mark Bricklin, "Journey to Health," *Prevention*, September, 1978, pp. 29–41. Also, Gris and Merlin, *op. cit.*, pp. 55–73.

22. Gris and Merlin, *op. cit.*, p. 323.

ADDITIONAL SOURCES

Dorothy A. Halpern, "Profile: Alexander A. Bogomolets," *American Review of Soviet Medicine*, December, 1943, vol. 1, no. 2, pp. 173–75.

W. C. McKain, "Observations on Old Age in the Soviet Union," *The Gerontologist*, 1967, vol. 7, no. 1.

Edward Podolsky, *Red Miracle: The Story of Soviet Medicine* (New York: Beechhurst Press, 1947).

Notes to Chapter 4: Longevity in the Mountains

1. Michael James, *The New York Times*, September 28, 1956.

2. David Davies, *The Centenarians of the Andes* (New York: Doubleday & Co., 1975), pp. 99–109.

3. *Ibid.*, p. 105.

4. *Ibid.*, p. 107.

5. *Ibid.*, p. 87.

6. *Ibid.*, pp. 113–24.

7. Grace Halsell, *Los Viejos* (Emmaus, Pa.: Rodale Press, 1976), p. 16.

8. *Ibid.*, p. 87.

9. *Ibid.*

10. *Ibid.*, p. 157.

11. An outstanding film that deals with old people in the Andes is *The Spirit Possession of Alejandro Mamani*, a documentary made by anthropologists in the Bolivian highlands. It deals with an 81-year-old Aymara Indian living under conditions similar to those in Vilcabamba. Although physically strong, Mamani is obsessed by the fear of evil spirits, illness, and abandonment. His paranoia eventually extends to distrusting his own relatives and friends, with financial concerns playing a role in his alienation. A grim epilogue to the film informs the viewer that after the anthropologists left the area, Alejandro Mamani committed suicide by leaping from a high cliff.

12. Alexander Leaf, *Youth in Old Age* (New York: McGraw-Hill, 1975) and Leaf, "Every Day Is a Gift When You Are over 100," *National Geographic*, January, 1973, vol. 143, no. 1, pp. 92–119.

13. Leaf, *Youth . . .*, p. 49.

14. Walter Sullivan, "Scientists Seek Key to Longevity," *The New York Times*, February 11, 1973, p. 1.

15. Richard B. Mazess and Sylvia H. Forman, "Longevity and Age Exaggeration in Vilcabamba, Ecuador, *Journal of Gerontology*, January, 1979, vol. 34, no. 1, pp. 94–98.

16. *Ibid.*, p. 97.

17. Walter Sullivan, "Very Old People in the Andes Are Found to Be Merely Old," *The New York Times*, March 17, 1978, p. 18.

18. International report summarized in Richard B. Mazess, "Health and Longevity in Vilcabamba, Ecuador," *Journal of the American Medical Association*, October 13, 1978, vol. 240, no. 16, p. 1781. Also see Mazess, "Bone Mineral in Vilcabamba, Ecuador," *American Journal of Roentgenology*, April, 1978, 130:671–74.

19. Wendell C. Bennet and Robert M. Zinge, *The Tarahumara* (Chicago: University of Chicago Press, 1935), pp. 349–50.

20. James Norman, "The Tarahumaras," *National Geographic*, May, 1976, vol. 149, no. 5, p. 717.

21. *Ibid.*, p. 717.

22. Henry Gris and Milton Merlin, *May You Live to Be 200!* (South Brunswick, N.J., and New York: A. S. Barnes, 1978).

23. Alexandru Ciuca, "Longevity and Environmental Factors," *The Gerontologist*, vol. 7, no. 4, pp. 252–56.

24. Suha Beller and Erdman Palmore, "Longevity in Turkey," *The Gerontologist*, October, 1974, vol. 14, no. 5, pp. 373–76.

25. J. N. Morris, J. A. Heady, et al., "Coronary Heart Disease and Physical Activity of Work," *Lancet*, 1953, 2:1053–57 and 1111–20.

26. M. J. Karvonen et al., "Longevity of Endurance Skiers," *Medicine and Science in Sports*, 1974, 6:49–56.

27. John Langone, *Long Life* (Boston: Little, Brown, 1978), p. 217.

28. Ralph S. Paffenbarger, Alvin L. Wing, and Robert T. Hyde, "Physical Activity as an Index of Heart Attack Risk in College Alumni," *American Journal of Epidemiology*, vol. 108, no. 3, September, 1978, pp. 161–75.

29. R. S. Paffenbarger, Jr., and W. E. Hales, "Work Activity and Coronary Heart Mortality," *New England Journal of Medicine*, 1975, 292:545. See also Ralph S. Paffenbarger, Mary Elizabeth Laughlin, Alfred S. Gima, and Rebecca A. Black, "Work Activity of Longshoremen as Related to Death from Coronary Heart Diseases and Stroke," *New England Journal of Medicine*, vol. 282, no. 20, May 14, 1970, pp. 1109–14.

30. J. N. Morris and M. D. Crawford, "Coronary Heart Disease and Physical Activity of Work. Evidence of a National Necropsy Survey," *British Medical Journal*, 1958, 2:1485–96, and J. N. Morris, C. Adam, S. Chave, et al., "Vigorous Exercise in Leisure Time and the Incidence of Coronary Heart Disease," *Lancet*, 1973, 1:333–39.

31. J. N. Morris, J. A. Heady, et al., *op. cit.*

ADDITIONAL SOURCES

Samuel M. Fox and John P. Naughton, "Physical Activity and the Prevention of Coronary Heart Disease," *Preventive Medicine*, 1972, I:92–120.

Harold A. Kahn, "The Relationship of Reported Coronary Heart Disease Mortality to Physical Activity of Work," *American Journal of Public Health*, 1963, 52: 1058-67.

Philip Sturgeon, Suha Beller, and Eleanor Bates, "Study of Blood Type Group Factors in Longevity," *Journal of Gerontology*, January, 1969, vol. 24, no. 1, pp. 90–94.

Henry Longstreet Taylor, Ernest Kleptear, Ancel Keys, et al., "Death Rates Among Physically Active and Sedentary Employees of the Railroad Industry," *American Journal of Public Health*, 1962, 52:1697–17007.

Notes to Chapter 5: The Hunzakuts

1. John Keay, *The Gilgit Game* (Hamden, Conn.: Archon, 1979) provides good background to the British exploration and seizure of Hunza.

2. Robert McCarrison, "Faulty Food in Relation to Gastro-Intestinal Disorder," Sixth Mellon Lecture delivered before the Society for Biological Research, University of Pittsburgh School of Medicine, November 18, 1921, 27 pages.

3. Firsthand accounts of the war appear in Col. Algernon Durand, *The Making of a Frontier* (London: Thomas Nelson, 1908) and in E. F. Knight, *Where Three Empires Meet* (London: Longman Green & Co., 1893). Dr. John Clark has informed the author by letter that in Nazim Khan's autobiography the Mir claimed to have withdrawn from a very strong position in order to ensure a British victory. The reward for his treachery was to take the place of his deposed brother. This is at odds with the British

accounts, which credit the Pathan troops for scaling a wall the defenders had thought unassailable.

4. Robert McCarrison, *Studies in Deficiency Diseases* (London: Henry Frowde and Hodder & Stoughton, 1921).

5. G. T. Wrench, *The Wheel of Health* (London: C. W. Daniel Co., Ltd., 1938).

6. J. I. Rodale, *The Healthy Hunzas* (Emmaus, Pa.: Rodale Press, 1949).

7. Jay Milton Hoffman, *Hunza* (Valley Center, Calif.: Professional Press Publishing Associates, 1968), p. 1.

8. Albert Abarbanel, "The Healthiest People in the World," *American Mercury*, September, 1954, pp. 43–44.

9. Allen Banik and Renee Taylor, *Hunza Land* (Long Beach, Calif.: Whitehorn Publishing Co., 1960).

10. James Hilton, *Lost Horizon* (New York: William Morrow & Co., 1933), p. 69.

11. E. O. Lorimer, *Language Hunting in the Karakoram* (London: George Allen & Unwin, Ltd., 1939).

12. Wilfred Skrede, *Across the Roof of the World* (New York: W. W. Norton, Inc., 1954).

13. John Clark, *Hunza: Lost Kingdom of the Himalayas* (London: Hutchinson & Co., 1957).

14. Jean Bowie Shor, *After You, Marco Polo* (New York: McGraw-Hill, 1955) and Jean and Frank Shor, "At World's End in Hunza," *National Geographic*, October, 1953, vol. CIV, no. 4, pp. 485–518.

15. Barbara Mons, *High Road to Hunza* (London: Faber & Faber, 1958).

16. Mellon Lecture, p. 10.

17. McCarrison, *op. cit.*, p. 9.

18. Robert McCarrison, "The Relationship of Diet to the Physical Efficiency of Indian Races," *The Practitioner* (London), January, 1925, pp. 90–100.

19. G. W. Leitner, *Results of a Tour in Dardistan, Kashmir, Little Tibet, Ladak, Zanskar, Etc. in 1866* (London: Trubner & Co., 1868–73), 4 volumes.

20. Major J. Biddulph, *Tribes of the Hindoo Koosh* (Calcutta: Office of the Superintendent of Government Printing, 1880).

21. John Clark, "Hunza in the Himalayas," *Natural History*, October, 1963, vol. LXXII, no. 6, pp. 38–46. Author also has corresponded with and phone-interviewed Dr. Clark in order to obtain additional data. Among Clark's comments were that goiter and cretinism were still rare in Hunza when he was there. He thought that goiter was just becoming common as the last residual iodine was being washed from the soil. He notes that appendicitis is generally absent in most parts of Asia except among people who have lived in the West.

22. Wrench, *op. cit.*, p. 101.

23. Mons, *op. cit.*, p. 104.

24. Alexander Leaf, *Youth in Old Age* (New York: McGraw-Hill, 1975), p. 37.

25. Wrench, *op. cit.*, p. 27.

26. McCarrison, "Relationship of Diet . . .," p. 95.

27. Lorimer, *op. cit.*, p. 184.

28. Telephone interview, 1979.

29. Mons, *op. cit.*, p. 106.

30. Walter R. Lawrence, *The Valley of Kashmir* (London: Henry Frowdie, 1895), p. 227.

31. Rodale, *op. cit.*, p. 200.

32. John Keay, *The Gilgit Game* contains numerous accounts. See also his excellent bibliography of nineteenth-century exploration of the area.

33. R. C. F. Schomberg, *Between the Oxus and the Indus* (London: Martin Hopkinson, Ltd., 1935), p. 137. Similar incident reported by McCarrison.

34. M. Auriel Stein, *Sand-Buried Ruins of Kohtan* (London: T. Fisher Unwin, 1903), p. 51. Similar incident reported by the Shors.

35. Sir Francis Younghusband, *Dawn in Asia* (London: John Murray, 1930), p. 192.

36. *Ibid.*, p. 174.

37. Leaf, *op. cit.*, p. 34.

38. Brian Jeffries, "Civilization Closing In on Shangri-La," *Los Angeles Times*, June 9, 1974, Section 8, p. 9, and "No More Shangri-La," *The Washington Post*, September 26, 1974, p. A10.

39. Audry Topping, "Opening a New Road to China: The Karakoram Highway," *The New York Times Magazine*, December 2, 1979, p. 136.

ADDITIONAL SOURCES

William Martin Conway, *Climbing and Exploration in Karakoram-Himalayas* (London: T. Fisher Unwin, 1894), four volumes.

George Curzon, *The Pamirs* (London: Royal Geographical Society, 1896).

Frederick Drew, *The Northern Barrier of India* (London: Edward Standford, 1877).

P. T. Etherton, *Across the Roof of the World* (London: Constable & Co., 1911).

The Pakistan Journal of Medical Research, April, 1966, has five medical articles on the health of the Hunzakuts, pp. 133–75.

George Scott Robertson, *The Kafirs of the Hindu-Kush* (London: Lawrence & Bullen, 1896).

R. C. F. Schomberg, *Unknown Karakoram* (London: Martin Hopkinson, Ltd., 1936).

Eric Shipton, *Mountains of Tartary* (London: Hodder & Stoughton, 1951).

H. M. Sinclair, *The Work of Robert McCarrison* (London: Faber & Faber, 1952). A collection of McCarrison's writings.

Renée Taylor as told to by His Highness Mir Mohd Jamal Khan, *Come Along to Hunza (The History of Shangri-La)* (Minneapolis: T. S. Denison & Co., 1974).

——— and Milford J. Nobbs, *Hunza: The Himalayan Shangri-La* (El Monte, California: Whiteman Publishing, 1962).

————, *Hunza Health Secrets for Long Life and Happiness* (Englewood Cliffs, N.J.: Prentice-Hall, 1964).

————, *The Hunza-Yoga Way to Health and Longer Life* (New York: Constellation International, 1969).

Lowell Thomas, *Book of the High Mountains* (New York: Julian Messner, Inc., 1964).

Jenny Visser-Hooft with contributions by P. C. Visser, *Among the Kara-Korum Glaciers in 1925* (London: Edward Arnold, 1926).

Notes to Chapter 6:
Serendipitous Sheringham and Cambridgeshire

1. "English Village Soil Linked To Longevity," *The New York Times*, October 6, 1977, p. 72, is typical.

2. 1971 Census of England and Wales, Norfolk Part I, Her Majesty's Stationery Office, 1973, pp. 18–27.

3. This and other interview material in the present chapter were obtained in September of 1978. All the centenarians discussed in the chapter had had their ages confirmed by a telegram from the Queen. This verification occurs when the claim of someone approaching 100 is brought to the attention of the Throne. The claim is then checked through official governmental records pertaining to that individual. If the age is valid, a telegram is sent on the appropriate birthday. The system, which involves the prestige of the Monarch, has established a record of reliability. Since none of the centenarians discussed in this chapter claimed an extreme age, the author did not think it necessary to independently verify their ages.

4. 1971 Census, *loc. cit.*

5. In addition to interview material, background on Mr. Cornelius is available in the files of the *Eastern Daily Press* and *North Norfolk News*. These were written from 1974 to 1979 at the time of his birthday.

6. A. Campbell Erroll, *A History of the Parishes of Sheringham and Beeston Regis* (Norwich: Rigby Printing Co., 1970) is his major work. Also: "Life and Death in Norfolk Villages," Part I—Sheringham typescript, Norwich Public Libraries, Local Collection, Norwich, and typescripts and other materials given to the author by A. Campbell Erroll.

7. "Life and Death in Norfolk Villages," Part III—A Village Community in 1791.

8. Author tabulated all deaths recorded in the church from 1800 to 1978.

9. Investigation made by author.

ADDITIONAL SOURCES

R. W. Apple, Jr., "Britain's Notable Nonagenarians," *The New York Times Magazine*, November 11, 1979, pp. 50–72.

All Saints Upper Sheringham, a pamphlet printed by Ashlock Magazine Center (Home Words, Ltd.), London, 1960.

Notes to Chapter 7:
Rethinking the First Ninety-Nine

1. Alexander Leaf, *Youth in Old Age*, (New York: McGraw-Hill, 1975), Introduction.

2. Alexander Leaf, "Getting Old," *Scientific American*, September, 1973, vol. 229, no. 3, pp. 45–52.

3. A vivid example of misdiagnosis can be seen in the film *The Last of Life*. Mr. and Mrs. Brown, previously diagnosed and institutionalized as "irreversibly demented," are shown talking with doctors and students after their recovery. Their "senility" was primarily a matter of overmedication, enforced separation because of an injury which hospitalized the husband, and depression. At the time the film was made, the couple had been reunited and were living independently. Twenty-eight-minute film from the Canadian Broadcasting Corporation.

4. Harvey Lehman, *Age and Achievement* (Princeton, N.J.: Princeton University Press, 1930) and Ruth A. Hubbell, "Men and Women Who Have Performed Distinctive Service After the Age of 74," *Wilson Bulletin for Librarians*, 1935, 9:297–305.

5. Sharon Johnson, "Welthy Fisher: Woman with a Mission," *The New York Times*, April 2, 1978, p. 54, and "Spreading the Word," *The New York Times*, September 18, 1979. Her autobiography is titled *To Light a Candle* (New York: McGraw-Hill, 1962).

6. Harold M. Schmeck, Jr., "Research Attempts to Fight Senility," *The New York Times*, July 31, 1979, and "Memory Loss Curbed by Chemical in Foods," *The New York Times*, January 9, 1979, p. C1.

7. Belle Boone Beard, "Some Characteristics of Recent Memory in Centenarians," *Journal of Gerontology*, January, 1968, vol. 23, no. 1, pp. 23–31. More general: Dr. Arthur S. Freese, *The End of Senility*, (New York: Arbor House, 1978) and Belle Boone Beard, *Social Competence of Centenarians* (Athens, Ga.: Social Science Research Institute, University of Georgia, 1967).

8. Harris Dienstfrey and Joseph Lederer, *What Do You Want to Be When You Grow Old?* (New York: Bantam, 1979), pp. 27–37. Cross-cultural references can be found in Robert Coles, *The Old Ones of New Mexico* (New York: Anchor/Doubleday, 1975) and Erdman Palmore, *The Honorable Elders* (Durham, N.C.: Duke University Press, 1975), a study of aging in Japan.

9. Stephen Jewett, "Longevity and the Longevity Syndrome," *The Gerontologist*, Spring, 1973, vol. 12, no. 1, pp. 91–99.

10. John Court, "Want to Live to Be 120?" *Atlas*, October, 1968, vol. 16, no. 4, pp. 54–55.

11. Herbert A. de Vries and Gene M. Adams, "Comparison of Exercise Responses in Old and Young Men," *Journal of Gerontology*, 1972, vol. 27, no. 3, and de Vries, "Prescription of Exercise for Older Men from Telemetered Exercise Heart Rate Data," *Geriatrics*, April, 1971.

12. Lewis *[sic]* Cornaro, *The Immortal Mentor* (Trenton, N.J.: Daniel Fenton, 1810).

13. Luigi Cornaro, *How to Live for a Hundred Years and Avoid Disease* (Oxford: Alden Press, 1935). Includes "Letter from a Nun of Padua" and *Spectator #105* by Addison.

14. Clive M. McCay, L. A. Maynard, et al., "Retarded Growth, Life Span, Ultimate Body Size and Age Changes in the Albino Rat After Feeding Diets Restricted in Calories," *Journal of Nutrition*, 1939, vol. 18, no. 1.

15. See discussion and citations in Nathaniel Altman, *Eating for Life* (Wheaton, Ill.: Theosophical Publishing House, 1977), pp. 21–23, 37.

16. One of the studies correlating wine consumption with heart disease is A. S. St. Leger, A. L. Cochrane, and F. Moore, "Factors Associated with Cardiac Mortality in Developed Countries with Particular Reference to the Consumption of Wine," *Lancet*, May 12, 1979, pp. 1017–20.

17. James Crichton-Browne, *The Doctor Remembers* (London: Ducksworth, 1938); A. Guéniot, *How to Live to Be a Hundred* (Valletta, Malta, 1933); and Hermann Weber, *On Longevity and the Means for the Prolongation of Life* (London: Macmillan & Co., 1939). Also useful: James Crichton-Browne, *The Prevention of Senility and a Sanitary Outlook* (London: Macmillan, 1905) and *Delusions in Diet* (London: Funk & Wagnalls, 1910).

18. Helen and Scott Nearing, *Living the Good Life* (New York: Schocken Books, Inc., 1970) and *Continuing the Good Life* (New York: Schocken Books, 1979).

19. A film has been made of the Nearings at their farm in Maine in which they discuss their way of life and the ideals that have molded it. It offers lively interviews full of good humor and views of their newly completed stone house. At the time of the film Scott was 93 and Helen was 73. *Living the Good Life*, produced by Bullfrog Films; thirty minutes. The film has won a number of awards.

20. The film, titled *Happy Birthday, Mrs. Craig*, has been shown on television. The centenarian speaks vigorously throughout the film, recalling the early days of black pioneers in the West. Equally notable are her continued advocacy of change and her relationship to her family, which numbers five generations. Produced by Richard Kaplan Productions, Inc.; one hour.

21. Sula Benet, *How to Live to Be 100* (New York: Dial Press, 1976) and in interview with the author.

22. Associated Press, "For More and More, Memories Span a Full Century," *The New York Times*, December 9, 1979, p. 67.

23. A higher theoretical life-span could be asserted on the basis that most animals live from 6 to 8 times as long as it takes them to reach maturity. Depending on whether one multiples by 6, 7, or 8 and at what age

maturity is reckoned, a span of 120 to 150 may be projected. This method is favored by those who would like to stretch the potential life-span far beyond anything ever reliably recorded and has so many scientific short-comings that it can be taken as only the roughest kind of guide.

ADDITIONAL SOURCES

Sir Richard Bulstrode, *Miscellaneous Essays* (London: John Browne, 1715) and *Letters* (London: R. Sare, 1712).
Alex Comfort, *A Good Age* (New York: Crown Press, 1976).
E. V. Cowdrey, *Aging Better* (Springfield, Ill.: Charles C. Thomas, 1972).
Robert S. De Ropp, *Man Against Dying* (New York: St. Martins Press, 1966).
Irene Gore, *Add Years to Your Life and Life to Your Years* (New York: Stein & Day, 1973).
Joan Gomez, *How Not to Die Young* (New York: Stein & Day, 1972).
W. Forbes Gray, *Five Score: A Group of Famous Centenarians* (London: John Murray, 1931).
Joel Kurtzman and Philip Gordon, *No More Dying* (Los Angeles: J. P. Tarcher, 1976).
Adrian M. Ostfeld and Don C. Gibson, editors, *Epidemiology of Aging*, Washington D.C., Department of Health, Education and Welfare Pub. No. (NIH) 75-711, 1972.
Charles Reinhardt, *120 Years of Life* (London: The London Publicity Co., 1910).
George Soule, *Longer Life* (New York: Viking, 1958).
Eric Weiser, *The Years in Hand* (New York: Abelard-Schuman, 1967).
Ruth Winter, *Ageless Aging* (New York: Crown, 1973).

Notes to Chapter 8: Doctor Two Legs

1. John T. Davis, *Walking* (New York: Bantam, 1979), pp. 85–87. A good introduction to the psychological and physiological benefits of walking.

2. Clarence M. Agress, *Energetics* (New York: Grosset & Dunlap, 1978).

3. Derek Clayton talks of forty-eight hours of urinating large clots of blood, persistent vomiting, and black diarrhea after running the world's fastest marathon. He states that it took him up to six months to fully recover. Richard Benyo, "Derek Clayton: The World's Fastest Marathoner," *Runner's World*, May, 1979, vol. 14, no. 5, pp. 66–73.

4. Desirable Weight Tables for Men and Women, Metropolitan Life Insurance Company, 1959. These are produced at intervals of approximately twenty years. As published the weights include indoor clothing and shoes. Following the system used by Kenneth Keyes in *How to Live*

Longer–Stronger–Slimmer (New York: Frederick Fell, Inc., 1966), the charts have been adapted to the nude body by subtracting 5 pounds of clothing for women (Metropolitan Life allows 2–4 pounds) and 8 pounds for men (Metropolitan Life allows 5–7). Heights are given for bare feet instead of one-inch heels for men and two-inch heels for women.

5. *Royal Canadian Air Force Exercise Plans for Physical Fitness* (New York: Bantam, 1972).

6. Kenneth H. Cooper, *Aerobics* (New York: Bantam, 1968).

7. John N. Leonard, J. L. Hofer, and N. Pritikin, *Live Longer Now* (New York: Grosset & Dunlap, 1974). Nathan Pritikin with Patrick M. McGrady, Jr., *The Pritikin Plan for Diet and Exercise* (New York: Grosset & Dunlap, 1979).

8. Truman Clark, "The Master's Movement," *Runner's World*, July, 1979, vol. 14, no. 7, pp. 80–95, has a number of charts showing running records for those from 40 to 100. Additional information on Iordanidis provided by Yannis Iordanidis from news clippings. Walking feats can be found in Davis, *Walking* and various other stunts by old people in the *Guinness Book of World Records*.

9. See Pritikin with McGrady, *op. cit.*, pp. 89–90, and Carol Lawson, "Behind the Best Sellers," *The New York Times*, July 1, 1979.

ADDITIONAL SOURCES

Grant Gwinup, *Energetics* (Los Angeles: Sherbourne Press, 1970).

Sir Percival Horton-Smith Hartley, "The Longevity of Oarsmen," *British Medical Journal*, April, 1939, vol. 1, p. 657.

C. Harley Hartung, John F. Foreyt, Robert E. Mitchell, et al., "Relation of Diet to High-Density-Lipoprotein Cholesterol in Middle-Aged Marathon Runners, Joggers, and Inactive Men," *New England Journal of Medicine*, vol. 302, no. 7, February 14, 1980, pp. 357–61.

Anthony P. Polednak, *The Longevity of Athletes* (Springfield, Ill.: Charles C. Thomas, 1979).

Yehuda Shoenfeld, Gad Keren, Tavia Shimoni, et al., "Walking—a Method for Rapid Improvement of Physical Fitness," *Journal of the American Medical Association*, 1980, 243:2062–63.

Notes to Chapter 9: Food as Fuel

1. Nathaniel Altman, *Eating for Life* (Wheaton, Ill.: Theosophical Publishing House, 1977) summarizes major vegetarian concepts.

2. Roland Phillips, "Role of Life-Style and Dietary Habits in Risk of Cancer Among Seventh-Day Adventists," *Cancer Research*, November, 1975, 35: 3513–22, does a very good job of factoring out influences of tobacco and tries to determine differences between those who have never

eaten meat, those who have quit, and those who continue to eat moderate amounts.

3. Some studies indicate that a B-12 deficiency can develop in vegetarians who eat no meat or dairy products. Vegans dispute this. See discussion in Altman, *op. cit.*, p. 150.

4. Interview by the author, 1978. Dinshah has been very skeptical of health claims tied to diets in places like Vilcabamba and Hunza. He has written an exposé and analysis of odd diets for his newspaper *Ahimsa* and reproduced it in packet form as *Fruit for Thought*. Available through American Vegan Society, Malaga, New Jersey.

5. Letitia Brewster and Michael F. Jacobson, *The Changing American Diet* (Washington D.C.: Center for Science in the Public Interest, 1978).

6. Altman, *op. cit.*, pp. 33–38, has extensive discussion and bibliography.

7. Joseph H. Highland, Marcia E. Fine, et al., *Malignant Neglect* (New York: Alfred A. Knopf, 1979), pp. 150–51, and Richard D. Lyons, "Chemical Tied to Cancer Is Banned as Cattle Feed," *The New York Times*, June 30, 1979, p. 6.

8. Highland et. al., *op cit.*, pp. 55–81.

9. "A Chemical Web of Contamination," *The New York Times*, December 19, 1979, C20; "PCB Contamination Is Reported in Food Produced in Four States," *The New York Times*, December 15, 1979; "66 Supermarkets Ban Eggs for High Levels of PCB," *The New York Times*, September 17, 1979, p. A1. Also see E. J. Dionne Jr., "State Drafts a Plan to Rid the Hudson of PCB 'Hot Spots,'" *The New York Times*, June 28, 1978, A1; and Richard Severo, "Efforts to Reduce PCB's in Food Stalled 3 Years After F.D.A. Vow," *The New York Times*, January 1, 1979, p. A1.

10. Iver Peterson, "Michigan PBB; Not a Comedy, but Plenty of Errors," *The New York Times*, July 2, 1978, p. E16, and "Farmers Shaken by Poison Case," *The New York Times*, August 8, 1979, p. A12.

11. "Salt and High Blood Pressure," *Consumer Reports*, March, 1979, pp. 147–49.

12. Easy-to-read summary in Jane E. Brody, "Personal Health: Alcohol Offers Some Benefits to Health as Well as Drawbacks," *The New York Times*, October 3, 1979. Also A. S. St. Leger, A. L. Cochrane, and F. Moore, "Factors Associated with Cardiac Mortality in Developed Countries with Particular Reference to the Consumption of Wine," *Lancet*, May 12, 1979, pp. 1017–20.

ADDITIONAL SOURCES

Clarence Agress, *Energetics* (New York: Grosset & Dunlap, 1978).

Charles H. Hennekins, B. Rosner, and D. S. Cole, "Daily Alcoholic Consumption and Fatal Coronary Heart Disease," *American Journal of Epidemiology* 107:1906–200, 1978.

Charles H. Hennekins, Walter Willet, Bernard Rosner, et al., "Effects of Beer, Wine, and Liquor in Coronary Deaths," *Journal of the*

American Medical Association, 242:1973–74, 1979. Contains a good section on additional sources. See also editorial in same issue.

William McQuade and Ann Aikman, *The Longevity Factor* (New York: Simon and Schuster, 1979).

Nevin S. Scrimsaw, "Protein Requirements—Strengths and Weaknesses of the Committee Approach," *New England Journal of Medicine,* vol. 29, no. 3, January 15, 1976, pp. 134–42, and vol. 29, no. 4, January 22, 1976, pp. 198–203 contain dissenting views on some aspect of the World Health Organization's recommendations, particularly in relation to young adults.

Notes to Chapter 10: Biochemical Individuality

1. Roger J. Williams, "Nutritional Individuality," *Human Nature,* June, 1978, vol. 1, no. 6, pp. 46–53.

2. Linus Pauling, *Vitamin C and the Common Cold* (San Francisco: W. H. Freeman and Co., 1970).

3. H. L. Newbold, *Vitamin C Against Cancer* (New York: Stein & Day, 1979) is very enthusiastic about the use of C in fighting diseases, particularly cancer. The book is most valuable in its transcripts of interviews with prominent physicians and researchers.

4. Newbold, *op. cit.,* includes a section on negative effects of megadoses of C in some patients and how to avoid those effects, as well as different forms of C and their effects. As an appendix it has the important study by Ewan Cameron and Linus Pauling, "Supplemental Ascorbate in the Supportive Treatment of Cancer: Prolongation of Survival Times in Terminal Human Cancer," originally published in *Proceedings* of the National Academy of Science, U.S.A., October, 1976, vol. 73, pp. 3685–89, Medical Science.

5. Priscilla W. Laws, *Medical and Dental X-Rays; A Consumer's Guide to Avoiding Unnecessary Radiation Exposure* (Washington, D.C.: Public Citizen, Health Research Group, 1974).

6. "Excess X-Ray Radiation Found," *The New York Times,* December 5, 1979, p. A12.

7. Harold Elrick, James Crakes, and Sam Clarke, *Living Longer and Better* (Mountain View, Calif.: World Publications, 1978), p. 153, and Hans J. Kugler, *Dr. Kugler's Seven Keys to a Longer Life* (New York: Stein & Day, 1978).

ADDITIONAL SOURCES

Ivan Illich, *Medical Nemesis* (London: Calder and Boyars, 1975).

Edward C. Lambert, *Modern Medical Mistakes* (Bloomington, Ind.: Indiana University Press, 1978).

Robert Mendelsohn, *Confessions of a Medical Heretic* (Chicago: Contemporary Books, 1979).

Recommended Dietary Allowances, 8th revised edition (Washington, D.C.: National Academy of Sciences, 1974).

Nathan W. Shock, editor, *Aging: Some Social & Biological Aspects* (Freeport, N.Y.: Books for Libraries Press, 1960).

Leonard Tushnet, *The Medicine Men* (New York: St. Martin's Press, 1971).

Notes to Chapter 11: The Longevous Personality

1. M. Friedman and R. H. Rosenman, *Type A Behavior and Your Heart* (New York: Alfred A. Knopf, 1974).

2. Hans Selye, *The Stress of Life* (New York: McGraw-Hill, 1976), revised edition.

3. The director and major researcher for the film, Idelfonso Ramos, was interviewed by the author after a screening of the film during a tour of U.S. film critics to Cuba in June, 1968. Inquiries about the film, which is not available in the United States at this writing, should be directed to the Cuban Film Institute, Havana, Cuba.

4. See discussion in Alex Comfort, *The Process of Ageing* (London: Weidenfeld & Nicolson, 1965), p. 69.

5. *Ibid.*, p. 67.

6. E. Pfeiffer, A. Verwoerdt, and H. S. Wang, "Sexual Behavior in Aged Men and Women," in E. Palmore, ed., *Normal Aging* (Durham, N.C.: Duke University Press, 1970). See also Gustave Newman and Claude R. Nichols, "Sexual Activities and Attitudes in Older Persons," *Journal of the American Medical Association,* 173:33–35, 1960, and Jane E. Brody, "Survey of Aged Reveals Liberal Views on Sex," *The New York Times,* April 22, 1980, p. C1.

7. Diana S. Woodruff, *Can You Live to Be 100?* (New York: Chatham Square Press, 1977), pp. 155–65.

8. Jules V. Quint and Bianca R. Cody, "Pre-eminence and Mortality: Longevity of Prominent Men," *The American Journal of Public Health,* vol. 60, no. 6, June, 1970, pp. 1118–24.

9. Metropolitan Life Insurance Company, "Longevity of Corporate Executives," *Statistical Bulletin,* 1974, 55:2–4.

10. G. Gallup and E. Hill, *The Secrets of Long Life* (New York: Bernard Geis Associates, 1960).

11. O. Carl Simonton, Stephanie Matthews-Simonton, and James Creighton, *Getting Well Again* (Los Angeles: J. P. Tarcher, Inc., 1978). A wider, equally informed view can be found in Kenneth R. Pelletier, *Mind as Healer, Mind as Slayer* (New York: Delacorte Press/Seymour Lawrence, 1977).

12. Norman Cousins, "What I Learned From 3,000 Doctors," reprinted from *The Saturday Review* in *Prevention,* June, 1978, vol. 30, no. 6, p. 109.

13. Norman Cousins, *Anatomy of an Illness* (New York: Norton, 1979).

14. Cousins, "What . . .," p. 109.

ADDITIONAL SOURCES

David Hendin, *Death as a Fact of Life* (New York: W. W. Norton & Co., 1973).

Brian Inglis, *The Case for Unorthodox Medicine.* (N.Y.: G.P. Putnam's Sons, 1965).

Gay Luce and Julius Segal, *Sleep* (New York: Coward-McCann, 1966).

Gustave Newman and Claude R. Nichols, "Sexual Activities and Attitudes in Older Persons," *Journal of the American Medical Association,* 1960, 173:33–35.

Nathaniel Weyl, "Survival Past the Century Mark," *Mankind Quarterly,* 1977, 17:163–65.

Notes to Chapter 12: The Toxic Society

1. Bayard Webster, "Acid Rain: An Increasing Threat," *The New York Times,* November 6, 1979, p. C1, is a good summary article. Webster describes the composition of the rain as follows: "Sulfur dioxide, which comprises about 60% of the acid components of the rains, is created almost entirely by the combustion of coal and oil in power plants, smelters, steel mills, factories, and space heaters. Nitrogen oxide, which makes up 35% of the acid in the rains, originates in the exhausts of internal combustion engines, mostly in automobiles, and in the emissions from high-temperature fossil fuel combustion." See also Alan J. Otten, "Industrial Countries Will Meet Next Week in Attempt to Curb Destructive Acid Rains," *The Wall Street Journal,* November 9, 1979.

2. Two excellent references to the multitude of problems involved are Samuel S. Epstein, *The Politics of Cancer* (San Francisco: Sierra Club Books, 1978) and Joseph H. Highland, Marcia E. Fine, et al., *Malignant Neglect* (New York: Alfred A. Knopf, 1979).

3. David Burnham, "Utility in Michigan Faces $450,000 Fine," *The New York Times,* November 10, 1979, p. 9.

4. Elizabeth Whelan, *Preventing Cancer* (New York: W. W. Norton & Co., Inc., 1978), pp. 52–76. See also David L. Levin, Susan S. Devesa, et al., *Cancer Rates and Risks* (Washington, D.C.: Department of Health, Education and Welfare Publication No. NIH 75-691).

5. Whelan, *op. cit.,* p. 213.

6. *Cancer Facts and Figures,* The American Cancer Society, 1977.

7. Harold Elrick, James Crakes, and Sam Clarke, *Living Longer and Better* (Mountain View, Calif.: World Publications, 1978), p. 182.

8. How this works in discouraging regulation of toxins and radiation can be seen in Harry Schwartz, "A Look at the Cancer Figures," *The Wall Street Journal,* November 15, 1979, editorial on p. 26.

9. Levin et al., *op. cit.,* p. 9.

10. Michael Phillips, "Lemon Tea Drinkers: A Group at Risk?" *New England Journal of Medicine*, 1979, 301:10005–6.

11. Quoted in *Energy Matters*, June, 1979, vol. 1, no. 2, p. 1.

12. Molly Ivins, "Denver Uncertain over Old Uranium Site," *The New York Times*, February 20, 1979, p. A13.

13. Howell Raines, "An Unwelcome Alabama Guest: Radioactive Gas in Many Homes," *The New York Times*, March 16, 1979, p. A1.

14. "Ex-Heads of Atomic Plant Admit Deliberate Release of Gases in '59," *The New York Times*, November 11, 1979, p. 63.

15. Molly Ivins, "Utah Uneasy over Leukemia–Atomic Tests Study," *The New York Times*, February 23, 1979. See also Joseph L. Lyon, Melville R. Klauber, John W. Gardner, and King, S. Udall, "Childhood Leukemia and Nuclear Fallout," *The New England Journal of Medicine*, 1979, 300:402–7. Editorial on the study in same issue.

16. Useful consumer guides for those concerned with possible water pollution are "Manual for Evaluating Public Drinking Water Supplies," available free from the Water Supply Division of the Environmental Protection Agency, Washington, D.C. 20460, and "Safe Drinking Water for All: What You Can Do," from League of Women Voters Education Fund, 25 cents.

ADDITIONAL SOURCES

Robert Alex Baron, *The Tyranny of Noise* (New York: St. Martin's Press, 1970).

Flaminio Cattebeni, Aldo Cavallaro, and Giovanni Galli, eds., *Dioxin: Toxicological and Chemical Aspects* (New York: Spectrum Publications, 1978).

Edwin Chen, *PBB: An Amercian Tragedy* (Englewood Cliffs, N.J.: Prentice-Hall, 1979).

Ron M. Linton, *Terracide* (Boston: Little, Brown & Co., 1970).

Notes to Chapter 13:
Redefining the Biological Limits

1. The best-known work of the group that calls itself the immortalists is Alan Harrington, *The Immortalist* (Millbrae, Calif.: Celestial Arts, 1969).

2. Albert Rosenfeld, *Prolongevity* (New York: Alfred A. Knopf, 1976).

3. Robert W. Prehoda, *Extended Youth* (New York: G. P. Putnam, 1968).

4. Patrick M. McGrady, Jr., *The Youth Doctors* (New York: Coward-McCann, 1968), pp. 53–58. An excellent survey of twentieth-century rejuvenation schemes.

5. Michel Gauguelin, *How Atmospheric Conditions Affect Your Health* (New York: Stein & Day, 1971).

ADDITIONAL SOURCES

Ernest Becker, *The Denial of Death* (New York: The Free Press–
Macmillan, 1973).
Victor Bogomoletz, *The Secret of Keeping Young* (London: Arco, 1954).
Daniel Hershey, *Lifespan* (Springfield, Ill.: Charles Thomas, 1964).
Saul Kent, *The Life-Extension Revolution* (New York: William Morrow,
1980).
Albert Krueger and David S. Sobel, "Air Ions & Health," in David S.
Sobel, ed., *Ways of Health* (New York: Harcourt Brace Jovanovich,
1979).
P. B. and J. S. Medawar, *The Life Science* (New York: Harper & Row,
1977).
Osborn Segerberg, Jr., *The Immortality Factor* (New York: E. P. Dutton,
1974).
Nathan W. Shock, ed., *Perspectives in Experimental Gerontology*
(Springfield, Ill.: Charles C. Thomas, 1966).
————, *Trends in Gerontology* (Stanford, Calif.: Stanford University Press,
1951).
Lee Weston, *Body Rhythm* (New York: Harcourt Brace Jovanovich, 1979).

Notes to Chapter 14: Longevity Now

1. W. G. Bowerman, "Centenarians," *Transactions* of the Actuary Society of America, 1939, 40:360–78; R. J. Myers, "Validity of Centenarian Data in the 1960 Census," *Demography*, 1966, 3:470–76; and "Centenarians," Metropolitan Life Insurance Co. Statistical Bulletin, 1971, pp. 3–4.

2. Jacob Siegel and Jeffrey S. Passel, "New Estimates of the Number of Centenarians in the U.S.," *Journal of the American Statistical Association*, September, 1976, vol. 71, no. 355, pp. 559–66.

3. "Few Gains Expected in Human Life Span," *The New York Times*, January 20, 1980, p. 44.

ADDITIONAL SOURCES

Herman Brotman, "Comparison of Life Expectancy, 1900 and 1974," *The
Gerontologist*, February, 1977, pp. 208–9.
Erdman Palmore and Frances C. Jeffers, *Prediction of Life Span*
(Lexington, Mass.: Heath Lexington Books, 1971).
Anthony Pearl and Ruth Dewitt Pearl, *The Ancestry of the Long-Lived*
(Baltimore: Johns Hopkins Press, 1934).

GLOSSARY

ACTUARY   An individual who computes insurance premiums on the basis of risk probabilities determined from statistical records.

AEROBIC   Utilizing oxygen.

ANOREXIA NERVOSA   A hysterical syndrome involving loss of appetite and aversion to food which can lead to deficiencies, emaciation, and even death.

ANTIOXIDANT   A substance which inhibits the conversion of an element into its oxide.

APPESTAT   The body's sense of appetite, a sense which can be highly influenced by psychological and cultural factors and which can be psychologically readjusted.

ARTERIOSCLEROSIS   A condition in which the walls of the arteries harden, thicken, and lose elasticity owing to mineral and fatty deposits.

ATHEROSCLEROSIS   The most common form of arteriosclerosis. A condition in which plaques containing cholesterol and fatty material build up on the inner lining of the arteries until they obstruct or block the flow of blood.

BASAL METABOLISM   The total of all chemical reactions within the body when it is resting in a fasting state.

BHA (butylated hydroxyanisole)   An antioxidant found in many processed foods or their packaging. It is considered safer than BHT but needs additional testing.

BHT (butylated hydroxytoluene)   An antioxidant used in many processed foods or their packaging. It may cause cancer and allergic reactions.

BIOLOGICAL AGING   The age of an organism indicated by its systemic fitness.

CARBOHYDRATES   A class of organic compounds required by the body for heat and energy which may also contain essential nutrients, such as vitamins and minerals.

CELLS   The structural units of all living things.

CENTENARIAN   Anyone at least 100 years of age.

CHOLESTEROL   An organic alcohol that is a universal tissue constituent. Found deposited in the vessel walls in atherosclerosis.

CHRONOLOGICAL AGE   The age of an organism indicated by the number of solar years it has existed.

DEVELOPED WORLD   Used in this book to indicate the United States, Canada, Europe, Japan, and all areas of the Soviet Union.

DIURETICS   Substances which stimulate an increase in the output of urine and thus temporarily cause loss of water in the body.

DNA (deoxyribonucleic acid)   A long string of atoms found in the nucleus of each cell. It controls all the characteristics of living things and transmits heredity.

ENZYMES   Proteins found in the cell which control most metabolic chemical reactions.

FATS   Foods composed of carbon, hydrogen, and oxygen which have more energy-producing power weight for weight than either carbohydrates or proteins.

FREE RADICALS   Unstable molecular fragments which last only a few thousandths of a second.

GENE   The unit of heredity transmitted in the chromosome.

GERIATRICS   A branch of medical science concerned with treating the diseases most prevalent among older people.

GERONTOLOGY   A branch of learning concerned with the study of aging in all its facets.

HORMONES   Chemical substances released into the bloodstream by the endocrine glands to stimulate body growth, resistance to stress, sexual functions, and other important bodily reactions.

IMMUNOLOGICAL SYSTEM   All those parts of the body which act to protect it from foreign substances.

LACTOVEGETARIAN   A vegetarian whose diet includes some dairy products.

LATE MATURITY   Used in this book to indicate persons who are at least 60 but have not reached 80 years of age.

LONGEVITY   Generally indicates great duration of life and in this book indicates a minimum age of 90 years.

MINERALS   Inorganic substances found in nature that are neither animal nor plant.

MINIMUM DAILY REQUIREMENT (MDR)   A standard developed by the Food and Drug Administration to indicate the daily amount of each identified essential nutrient which prevents symptoms of an actual deficiency disease in most persons.

NONAGENARIAN   Any person over the age of 90 but not yet 100 years of age.

OLD   In this book indicates a person more than 80 but not yet 90 years of age.

PHAGOCYTE   A blood cell that destroys foreign particles, bacteria, and cells.

PITUITARY   A small endocrine gland located at the base of the skull.

PLACEBO   A pill, injection, or other treatment containing no active medication.

PLACEBO EFFECT   A physical reaction resulting from a placebo.

PROLONGEVOUS   Used as an adjective to indicate something which favors longevity and used as a noun to indicate persons who consciously plan for long life.

PROTEINS   Nitrogenous organic compounds essential to bodily growth and maintenance.

RECOMMENDED DAILY ALLOWANCE (RDA)   A standard established by the National Academy of Sciences to indicate the amount of a known nutrient needed by a healthy person. This standard is used to help determine the United States Recommended Daily Allowances (USRDA), a value used for nutritional labeling by the Food and Drug Administration. The USRDA uses higher estimates of nutritional needs than the RDA because it is to be used as a guideline by the general population.

RNA (ribonucleic acid)   A long chain of atoms produced by the DNA to direct the formation of proteins.

SENILITY   A vague term with no precise scientific measure which generally refers to decaying mental ability.

SOMATYPE   Bodily shape.

SUPERCENTENARIAN   Used in this book to indicate anyone over 115 years of age.

SUPERLONGEVOUS   Used in this book to indicate anyone over the age of 110 but less than 115 years of age.

SYNDROME   A group of symptoms that characterizes a particular condition.

TRACE ELEMENT   A mineral required by the body in minute quantities.

TRIGLYCERIDE   A major storage form of fatty acids, and the major constituent of fatty tissue.

VEGAN   A "pure" vegetarian whose diet excludes all animal products (milk, cheese, eggs, and so on) with the exception of human milk for infants.

VITAMINS   Organic compounds needed for growth and life maintenance.

INDEX

333